T0264176

Orthopedic Anesthesiology

Editors

NABIL M. ELKASSABANY
EDWARD R. MARIANO

ANESTHESIOLOGY CLINICS

www.anesthesiology.theclinics.com

Consulting Editor
LEE A. FLEISHER

December 2014 • Volume 32 • Number 4

ELSEVIER

1600 John F. Kennedy Boulevard • Suite 1800 • Philadelphia, Pennsylvania, 19103-2899

http://www.theclinics.com

ANESTHESIOLOGY CLINICS Volume 32, Number 4
December 2014 ISSN 1932-2275, ISBN-13: 978-0-323-32638-4

Editor: Jennifer Flynn-Briggs
Developmental Editor: Susan Showalter

Anesthesiology Clinics (ISSN 1932-2275) is published quarterly by Elsevier Inc., 360 Park Avenue South, New York, NY 10010-1710. Months of issue are March, June, September, and December. Periodicals postage paid at New York, NY and at additional mailing offices. Subscription prices are $160.00 per year (US student/resident), $330.00 per year (US individuals), $400.00 per year (Canadian individuals), $533.00 per year (US institutions), $674.00 per year (Canadian institutions), $225.00 per year (Canadian and foreign student/resident), $455.00 per year (foreign individuals), and $674.00 per year (foreign institutions). To receive student and resident rate, orders must be accompanied by name of affiliated institution, date of term, and the *signature* of program/residency coordinator on institutions letterhead. Orders will be billed at individual rate until proof of status is received. Foreign air speed delivery is included in all *Clinics'* subscription prices. All prices are subject to change without notice. POSTMASTER: Send address changes to *Anesthesiology Clinics,* Elsevier Health Sciences Division, Subscription Customer Service, 3251 Riverport Lane, Maryland Heights, MO 63043. Customer Service (orders, claims, online, change of address): Elsevier Health Sciences Division, Subscription Customer Service, 3251 Riverport Lane, Maryland Heights, MO 63043. Tel: 1-800-654-2452 (U.S. and Canada); 314-447-8871 (outside U.S. and Canada). Fax: 314-447-8029. E-mail: journalscustomerservice-usa@elsevier.com (for print support); journalsonlinesupport-usa@elsevier.com (for online support).

Reprints. For copies of 100 or more of articles in this publication, please contact the Commercial Reprints Department, Elsevier Inc., 360 Park Avenue South, New York, NY 10010-1710. Tel.: 212-633-3874; Fax: 212-633-3820; E-mail: reprints@elsevier.com.

Anesthesiology Clinics, is also published in Spanish by McGraw-Hill Inter-americana Editores S. A., P.O. Box 5-237, 06500 Mexico D. F., Mexico.

Anesthesiology Clinics, is covered in *MEDLINE/PubMed (Index Medicus)*, *Current Contents/Clinical Medicine*, *Excerpta Medica*, *ISI/BIOMED*, and *Chemical Abstracts*.

Contributors

CONSULTING EDITOR

LEE A. FLEISHER, MD
Robert D. Dripps Professor and Chair of Anesthesiology & Critical Care; Professor of Medicine, Perelman School of Medicine, University of Pennsylvania, Philadelphia, Pennsylvania

EDITORS

NABIL M. ELKASSABANY, MD, MSCE
Assistant Professor and Director, Section of Orthopedic Anesthesiology, Department of Anesthesiology and Critical Care, Perelman School of Medicine, University of Pennsylvania, Philadelphia, Pennsylvania

EDWARD R. MARIANO, MD, MAS (Clinical Research)
Chief, Anesthesiology and Perioperative Care Service and Associate Chief of Staff, Inpatient Surgical Services, VA Palo Alto Health Care System, Palo Alto; Associate Professor, Department of Anesthesiology, Perioperative and Pain Medicine, Stanford University School of Medicine, Stanford, California

AUTHORS

RICHARD B. ABEL, MD
Instructor in Anesthesiology, Department of Anesthesiology, The Icahn School of Medicine at Mount Sinai Medical Center, New York, New York

OMAR I. AHMED, MD
Senior Instructor, Department of Anesthesiology and Critical Care Medicine, Johns Hopkins University School of Medicine, Baltimore, Maryland

JAIMO AHN, MD, PhD
Department of Orthopedic Surgery, Perelman School of Medicine, University of Pennsylvania, Philadelphia, Pennsylvania

JAIME L. BARATTA, MD
Clinical Assistant Professor of Anesthesiology, Department of Anesthesiology, Thomas Jefferson University, Philadelphia, Pennsylvania

LAURA CLARK, MD
Professor, Department of Anesthesiology and Perioperative Medicine, Residency Program Director, Director of Regional Anesthesia and Acute Pain, University of Louisville School of Medicine, Louisville, Kentucky

OSCAR A. DE LEONCASASOLA, MD
Chief, Division of Pain Medicine, Professor of Anesthesiology and Medicine, Vice-chair for Clinical Affairs, Department of Anesthesiology, Professor of Oncology, Roswell Park Cancer Institute, University at Buffalo, Buffalo, New York

NABIL M. ELKASSABANY, MD, MSCE
Assistant Professor, Director; Section of Orthopedic Anesthesiology, Department of Anesthesiology and Critical Care, Perelman School of Medicine, University of Pennsylvania, Philadelphia, Pennsylvania

KISHOR GANDHI, MD, MPH, CPE
Staff Anesthesiologist, Department of Anesthesiology, University Medical Center of Princeton, Plainsboro Township, New Jersey

NEIL A. HANSON, MD
Staff Anesthesiologist, Department of Anesthesiology, Virginia Mason Medical Center, Seattle, Washington

JAMES HITT, MD, PhD
Assistant Professor of Anesthesiology, Department of Anesthesiology, University at Buffalo, Buffalo, New York

REBECCA L. JOHNSON, MD
Assistant Professor of Anesthesiology, College of Medicine, Mayo Clinic, Rochester, Minnesota

T. EDWARD KIM, MD
Director of Acute Pain Medicine and Regional Anesthesiology, Anesthesiology and Perioperative Care Service, VA Palo Alto Health Care System, Palo Alto; Clinical Assistant Professor (Affiliated), Department of Anesthesiology, Perioperative and Pain Medicine, Stanford University School of Medicine, Stanford, California

SANDRA L. KOPP, MD
Associate Professor of Anesthesiology, College of Medicine, Mayo Clinic, Rochester, Minnesota

JIABIN LIU, MD, PhD
Department of Anesthesiology and Critical Care, Perelman School of Medicine, University of Pennsylvania, Philadelphia, Pennsylvania

DANIELLE B. LUDWIN, MD
Associate Professor of Anesthesiology, Division of Regional and Orthopedic Anesthesia, Department of Anesthesiology, Columbia University College of Physicians & Surgeons, New York, New York

MARCHYARN MAHATHANARUK, DO
Fellow in Pain Medicine, Department of Anesthesiology, University at Buffalo, Buffalo, New York

EDWARD R. MARIANO, MD, MAS (Clinical Research)
Chief, Anesthesiology and Perioperative Care Service and Associate Chief of Staff, Inpatient Surgical Services, VA Palo Alto Health Care System, Palo Alto; Associate Professor, Department of Anesthesiology, Perioperative and Pain Medicine, Stanford University School of Medicine, Stanford, California

STAVROS G. MEMTSOUDIS, MD, PhD, FCCP
Department of Anesthesiology, Hospital for Special Surgery, Weill Medical College of Cornell University, New York, New York

RAINHOLD ORTMAIER, MD
Department of Trauma Surgery and Sports Traumatology, Paracelsus Medical University, Salzburg, Austria

MARJORIE ROBINSON, MD
Assistant Professor, Department of Anesthesiology and Perioperative Medicine, Pain Fellowship Director, University of Louisville School of Medicine, Louisville, Kentucky

MEG A. ROSENBLATT, MD
Professor of Anesthesiology and Orthopedics, Department of Anesthesiology, The Icahn School of Medicine at Mount Sinai Medical Center, New York, New York

FRANCIS V. SALINAS, MD
Staff Anesthesiologist, Department of Anesthesiology, Virginia Mason Medical Center, Seattle, Washington

ERIC S. SCHWENK, MD
Assistant Professor of Anesthesiology, Department of Anesthesiology, Thomas Jefferson University, Philadelphia, Pennsylvania

OTTOKAR STUNDNER, MD
Department of Anesthesiology, Perioperative Medicine and Intensive Care Medicine, Paracelsus Medical University, Salzburg, Austria

BENJAMIN A. VAGHARI, MD
Assistant Professor, Department of Anesthesiology and Critical Care Medicine, Johns Hopkins University School of Medicine, Baltimore, Maryland

MARINA VARBANOVA, MD
Assistant Professor, Department of Anesthesiology and Perioperative Medicine, Director of Anesthesia VA Hospital, University of Louisville School of Medicine, Louisville, Kentucky

EUGENE R. VISCUSI, MD
Professor of Anesthesiology, Department of Anesthesiology, Thomas Jefferson University, Philadelphia, Pennsylvania

CHRISTOPHER L. WU, MD
Professor, Department of Anesthesiology and Critical Care Medicine, Johns Hopkins University School of Medicine, Baltimore, Maryland

Contents

usually older, with significant comorbidities. Delayed surgical treatment beyond 48 hours after admission is associated with significantly higher mortality. Hereby clinicians are presented with the challenge to optimize the complex hip fracture within a short time period. This article reviews the evidence regarding preoperative, intraoperative, and postoperative considerations, and provides insights into the best strategies with which to optimize the patient's condition and improve perioperative outcomes.

The basic principles of perioperative immune function with regard to cancer recurrence and infection are reviewed. The role of regional anesthesia-analgesia in preservation of immune function and available published data are discussed.

With the anticipated increase in the number of total joint arthroplasty surgeries and associated fall risks, a fall reduction program can provide greater safety for patients in the postoperative period. Although further prospective studies are needed among total joint arthroplasty patients, there is sufficient evidence to show that a successful fall reduction program can be implemented. Common components to date have included a multidisciplinary team, multicomponent interventions specific to the risks associated with total knee and hip arthroplasty patients, education of patients and staff, and strategies to promote adherence to the program.

Clinical pathways for total joint arthroplasty have been shown to reduce costs and significantly impact perioperative outcomes mainly through reducing provider variability. Effective clinical pathways link evidence to individual practice and balance costs with local experience, outcomes, and access to resources for responsible perioperative management. Common components of clinical pathways with major impact on perioperative outcomes are: 1) implementing pathways designed to include multimodal analgesia with regional anesthesia, 2) use of tranexamic acid to reduce blood loss, and 3) preconditioning followed by participation in early, accelerated rehabilitation programs to prevent postoperative complications related to immobility.

Orthopedic patients frequently have multiple comorbidities when they present for surgery. This article discusses risk stratification of this population and the preoperative work-up for patients with specific underlying conditions who often require orthopedic procedures. Preoperative strategies to decrease exposure to allogeneic blood and advantages of the Perioperative Surgical Home model in this unique population are discussed.

Successful implementation of an acute pain management service involves a team approach in which team members have clearly defined roles. Clinical protocols are designed to help address common problems and prevent errors. As the complexity of surgery and patients' diseases continues to increase, current knowledge of new analgesic medications, acute pain literature, and skills in regional anesthesia techniques is imperative. Emphasizing a multimodal approach can improve analgesia and decrease opioid-related side effects.

This article presents an overview of how to set up an ambulatory regional anesthesia program for orthopedic surgery. This information is valuable to anesthesiologists who want to expand their regional anesthesia practice and provides a greater understanding of relevant issues and strategies to maximize success.

The prevalence of opioid use in the North America and some countries of the European Union has resulted in an increase in the number of patients who may exhibit opioid tolerance when requiring postoperative pain management. The approach to postoperative pain control in these patients is different from the strategies used in opioid-naïve patients. Better understanding of the cellular mechanisms of opioid tolerance in animals has resulted in the transfer of these concepts from the basic research to the clinical arena. This article presents new developments in opioid tolerance and how this knowledge can be applied to clinical practice.

ANESTHESIOLOGY CLINICS

Foreword

Orthopedic Anesthesia

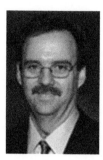

Lee A. Fleisher, MD
Consulting Editor

In the context of health care reform, it is increasingly important for anesthesiologists to demonstrate their value in patient care. One of the areas that has received a great deal of attention in that anesthesiologists impact the quality and costs of care is in orthopedic surgery. With the development of regional anesthesia and increasing interest in assessing outcomes after orthopedic surgery, anesthesiologists have taken a leadership role in delivering value. Much of the success of the Perioperative Surgical Home is in the area of orthopedic anesthesia. In this issue of *Anesthesiology Clinics*, a selection of excellent articles highlights the care paradigms and outcomes in this population.

In choosing guest editors for this issue, I solicited Nabil M. Elkassabany, MD, MSCE, Assistant Professor of Anesthesiology and Critical Care at the University of Pennsylvania Perelman School of Medicine, and Edward R. Mariano, MD, MAS, Associate Professor of Anesthesiology at Stanford University School of Medicine. Dr Mariano is also Chief of Anesthesiology and Perioperative Care Service and Associate Chief of Staff for the Inpatient Surgical Services. Both of these individuals have led Divisions of Regional Anesthesia and have formal training in clinical research and therefore have the expertise to ensure that the care paradigms are both evidence-based and lead to better outcomes. Both of them have also published original articles and reviews in the area of regional anesthesia and orthopedic surgery. Together they have solicited an outstanding group of contributors, including themselves, to provide us with the most up-to-date information.

Lee A. Fleisher, MD
Perelman School of Medicine
University of Pennsylvania
Philadelphia, PA 19104, USA

E-mail address:
Lee.fleisher@uphs.upenn.edu

Anesthesiology Clin 32 (2014) xi
http://dx.doi.org/10.1016/j.anclin.2014.09.002
1932-2275/14/$ – see front matter © 2014 Elsevier Inc. All rights reserved.

Preface

Orthopedic Anesthesia

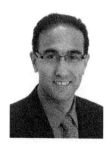 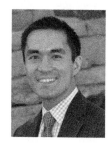

Nabil M. Elkassabany, MD, MSCE   Edward R. Mariano, MD, MAS (Clinical Research)
Editors

The practice of orthopedic anesthesiology has evolved over the past two decades to encompass many different orthopedic surgery service lines. The practice of the subspecialty is naturally diverse and covers all aspects of the perioperative continuum of care. The skill set required by the modern orthopedic anesthesiologist ranges from caring for geriatric patients with multiple comorbidities presenting urgently for operative repair of femur fractures, or electively for joint replacement, to caring for young healthy individuals presenting for a variety of sports injuries or trauma. Practice settings run the gamut from ambulatory surgery centers to inpatient care in intensive care units. Orthopedic anesthesiologists often use regional anesthesia techniques and may lead acute pain medicine services or get involved with hospital administration in setting up clinical care pathways. In many ways, orthopedic anesthesiologists are poised to lead in modeling the perioperative surgical home initiative promoted by the American Society of Anesthesiologists.

Given this diversity in practice and many recent advances in the field, we have dedicated this issue of *Anesthesiology Clinics* to present topics and updates specifically in orthopedic anesthesiology. This issue serves as a comprehensive evidence-based manual of orthopedic anesthesiology that can be used regularly for reference whenever clinical or systems-based challenges arise in practice. This compilation of articles addresses many frequently asked questions related to preoperative evaluation, setting up acute pain service, and setting up an ambulatory regional anesthesia program. Also included are tips and strategies for caring for orthopedic trauma patients or those with chronic opioid use. Some of the articles included in this issue provide suggestions for designing protocols for falls prevention and the perioperative management of patients presenting for repair of hip fractures or total joint arthroplasty. In addition, we have included timely topics, such as the latest evidence on how regional anesthesia may affect cancer recurrence, infection, and inflammation, and the evidence to support the use of ultrasound in the practice of regional anesthesia.

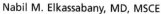

Anesthesiology Clin 32 (2014) xiii–xiv
http://dx.doi.org/10.1016/j.anclin.2014.09.001
1932-2275/14/$ – see front matter © 2014 Published by Elsevier Inc.

We are excited to have such an illustrious group of experts from around the United States contributing to this issue, sharing their experience, and discussing up-to-date evidence-based strategies to tackle key questions about orthopedic anesthesia. We are so grateful for their willingness to share their experience and for donating their time and effort. We also wish to thank our spouses and families for their unconditional and relentless support.

Nabil M. Elkassabany, MD, MSCE
Section of Orthopedic Anesthesiology
Department of Anesthesiology and Critical Care
Perelman School of Medicine, University of Pennsylvania
Philadelphia, PA 19104, USA

Edward R. Mariano, MD, MAS (Clinical Research)
Anesthesiology and Perioperative Care Service
Inpatient Surgical Services
Veterans Affairs Palo Alto Health Care System
Department of Anesthesiology, Perioperative
and Pain Medicine
Stanford University School of Medicine
Stanford, CA, USA

E-mail addresses:
Nabil.Elkassabany@uphs.upenn.edu (N.M. Elkassabany)
emariano@stanford.edu (E.R. Mariano)

Evidence-Based Medicine for Ultrasound-Guided Regional Anesthesia

Francis V. Salinas, MD*, Neil A. Hanson, MD

KEYWORDS

- Ultrasound guidance • Peripheral nerve blocks • Central neuraxial blocks
- Complications • Peripheral nerve injury • Local anesthetic systemic toxicity

KEY POINTS

- Ultrasound guidance (USG) has had a profound effect on regional anesthesiology and acute pain medicine.
- Despite the heterogeneity in the design of multiple randomized controlled trials, USG has consistently provided improved outcomes regarding block procedure time, block onset time, and (depending on the varying definitions) increased block success for single-injection and continuous peripheral nerve blocks.
- More recent data support a role for preprocedural USG in patients with predictors of technically difficult spinal anesthesia.
- Although the evidence for decreasing the risk of peripheral injury is currently lacking, accumulating evidence confirms that USG decreases but (just as important) does not eliminate the risk of local anesthetic systemic toxicity.
- The focus of research has appropriately changed to investigating the optimal USG techniques for specific nerve blocks and emerging data should further expand the applications and benefits of regional anesthesia.

INTRODUCTION

Ultrasound guidance (USG) has gained widespread acceptance in anesthesiology and perioperative medicine.[1,2] Evidence strongly supports increased safety, effectiveness, and efficiency of vascular access with USG compared with anatomic landmark-based techniques.[3] Regional anesthesia, especially for peripheral nerve blocks (PNBs), has increased in popularity during the last decade primarily due to the widespread adoption of USG as the dominant technique for nerve localization. In 2010, The American Society of Regional Anesthesia and Pain Medicine published an executive summary and

The authors have no financial conflicts of interest to disclose.
Department of Anesthesiology, Virginia Mason Medical Center, 1100 9th Avenue, Mailstop B2-AN, Seattle, WA 98101, USA
* Corresponding author.
E-mail address: Francis.salinas@vmmc.org

Anesthesiology Clin 32 (2014) 771–787
http://dx.doi.org/10.1016/j.anclin.2014.08.001
1932-2275/14/$ – see front matter © 2014 Elsevier Inc. All rights reserved.

accompanying series of articles, providing evidenced-based recommendations on the use of USG for regional anesthesia.[4-9] This series of articles critically appraised outcomes (**Box 1**) comparing USG to traditional landmark-based techniques (predominantly peripheral nerve stimulation [PNS]) as a nerve localization tool. Central to this series was the inclusion of only randomized controlled trials (RCTs), systematic reviews, meta-analyses, comparative studies, and large case series investigating the specific primary outcomes (see **Box 1**). Overall, these articles demonstrated that, for PNBs, USG provided a more rapid onset of sensory and/or motor block, increased block success, improved block quality (sensory and/or motor), decreased block performance time, and decreased local anesthetic dose requirements.[4-9] Almost all studies did not specifically investigate or were not powered for success of surgical anesthesia as the primary outcome. At that time, there was insufficient evidence demonstrating a decrease in the incidence of clinically relevant patient-safety outcomes of peripheral nerve injury (PNI), local anesthetic systemic toxicity (LAST), or pneumothorax. Notably, there was a lack of published data directly comparing USG to traditional landmark-based techniques for central neuraxial anesthesia. Two subsequent meta-analyses specifically investigated the primary outcome measure of anesthesia sufficient for surgery without supplementation (additional nerve blocks or exceeding a predetermined amount of intravenous systemic analgesia) or conversion to general anesthesia. The pooled data from these 2 meta-analyses showed that USG was associated with an increased success rate of surgical block.[10,11] However, caution is warranted when interpreting the results from these pooled data because surgical anesthesia was not the primary outcome in almost all of the individual RCTs in these meta-analyses.

Box 1
Outcome variables examined in ultrasound-guided regional anesthesia

- Block performance time (imaging and needle-guidance times)
- Successful placement and success of quality of CPNBs
- Number of needle passes and redirections
- Patient comfort during block placement
- Block onset
- Anesthesia-related time (performance and onset times)
- Local anesthetic requirements
- Block success (predefined quality of block within a specified timeframe)
  - Density of sensory block
  - Density of motor block
  - Surgical anesthesia without need for conversion to general (spinal) anesthesia or supplemental (systemic analgesics or additional nerve blocks)
- Complications
  - Vascular puncture (injury)
  - Peripheral nerve injury
  - Pneumothorax
  - Hemidiaphragmatic paresis
  - Local anesthetic systemic toxicity
- Cost-effectiveness

After this series of articles, there has been a paucity of RCTs directly comparing USG to PNS for PNBs. There are several reasons: (1) USG has rarely been found to be inferior to PNS, so perhaps there is less interest in adding additional data regarding the benefits of USG compared with PNS; (2) with the rapid improvement (increased image quality and portability) and decreased cost of ultrasound (US) technology, the cost-benefit argument against USG continues to decrease in terms of economic relevance; (3) the widespread adoption of USG as the dominant technique of peripheral nerve localization[12,13]; and (4) a shift in the emphasis on future research defining the optimal techniques for USG regional anesthesia.[14,15] The latter is reflected in the number of lectures and workshops dedicated specifically to USG (and few, if any, on PNS) at national and international meetings with a focus on regional anesthesia, as well as the shift in priority to education and training in USG regional anesthesia.[16,17] This article attempts to summarize and critically assess any additional data in the last 5 years directly comparing USG to PNS, including outcomes data for the use of USG for continuous PNBs (CPNBs). More specifically, due to the rare incidence of serious complications (PNS, LAST, and pneumothorax) and the lack of power of individual RCTs to demonstrate a statistically significant difference,[9] the authors provide a critical assessment of recently published large databases and registries providing, when available, the most recent point estimates of the risk of these rare complications. The authors also critically assess more recent data regarding the optimal techniques for USG PNBs, and more recent data from RCTs regarding the potential outcome benefits of USG for spinal anesthesia.

REVIEW OF MORE RECENT EVIDENCE DIRECTLY COMPARING ULTRASOUND GUIDANCE TO PERIPHERAL NERVE STIMULATION FOR PERIPHERAL NERVE BLOCKS

Two recent RCTS examined block performance times directly comparing USG to PNS in anesthesia trainees.[18,19] In a study of 41 subjects undergoing preoperative interscalene block before arthroscopic shoulder surgery, USG resulted in a statistically significant decrease in block performance time of 57% (4.3 ± 1.5 vs 10 ± 1.5 minutes) and sensory block onset time of 37% (12 ± 2 vs 19 ± 2 minutes).[18] There was no difference in block success for surgical anesthesia, which was similarly high in both groups (95% vs 91%), most likely due to the large mass of local anesthetic (300 mg mepivacaine and 150 mg ropivacaine in 40 mL volume) used in this protocol. In a study of 71 subjects undergoing hallux valgus repair using popliteal sciatic nerve block (PSNB), USG (with targeted circumferential injection around the tibial nerve [TN] and common peroneal nerve [CPN]) did not provide any increase in onset time or surgical block success (94% in both groups) within 30 minutes compared with PNS (eliciting both TN and CPN evoked motor responses [EMRs]).[19] USG decreased block performance time by 20% (82 seconds), although this was a secondary outcome.

In 60 subjects scheduled for upper limb surgery (at or distal to the elbow) undergoing preoperative infraclavicular block (ICB), subjects were randomized to either USG (5 mL bupivacaine 0.5% at each of the lateral, posterior, and medial cords) or PNS (accepting triceps or intrinsic hand muscle EMRs with the 15 mL volume of bupivacaine 0.5% injected). This was powered to detect a 10-minute difference in complete sensory and motor block onset.[20] There was no significant difference in block procedure time (likely reflecting the need for multiple redirections targeting all three cords in the US group vs a single EMR with PNS) or block onset time. Although, it was a secondary outcome, USG resulted in a 100% block success at 30 minutes compared with 74% with PNS. In a study of 52 subjects undergoing PSNB block before hallux valgus repair, subjects were randomized to either USG (short-axis out-of-plane approach at the sciatic bifurcation targeting the TN and CPN branches) or PNS (accepting a plantar-flexion EMR) with 20 mL mepivacaine 1.5%.[21] The proportion of subjects with a complete sensory (80% vs 4%) and motor block (60% vs 8%) at 15 minutes was significantly higher with USG, although by 30 minutes all subjects had adequate sensory block to allow surgery without supplementation. In 39 subjects undergoing interscalene block with ropivacaine 0.5% before arthroscopic shoulder surgery under general anesthesia, the minimum effective anesthetic volume (MEAV) required to achieve a postoperative verbal rating scale of 0 was compared for USG and PNS.[22] The MEAV required to provide effective analgesia was lower with USG (0.9 mL, 95% CI 0.3–2.8 vs 5.4 mL, 95% CI 3.4–8.6). Despite this difference, it is notable that the MEAV for effective postoperative analgesia was relatively low (<10 mL) in both groups. In the most recent RCT directly comparing USG to PNS in subjects receiving interscalene block for shoulder surgery, there was no difference in sensory block onset time (required for surgical anesthesia) using 20 mL of ropivacaine 1%.[23] Because studies have shown that successful interscalene brachial plexus block with USG may be achieved with much lower doses of ropivacaine (7 mL ropivacaine 0.75%),[24,25] any differences potentially provided by USG in this trial were very likely masked by the use of a relatively large total dose of local anesthetic in both groups.

REVIEW OF MORE RECENT EVIDENCE FOR ULTRASOUND GUIDANCE IN CENTRAL NEURAXIAL ANESTHESIA

Based on the limited evidence available at the time of the initial evidence-based review,[8] no firm recommendations were provided, although it was suggested that USG for central neuraxial anesthesia may be a useful adjunct to traditional landmark-based physical examination. The current application of USG for central neuraxial block may be classified into 2 categories: (1) US-assisted technique and (2) real-time USG technique.

Ultrasound-Assisted Technique

Two complementary scanning planes are used to identify acoustic windows for subsequent needle insertion and advancement: a transverse-midline (TM) plane and a paramedian sagittal-oblique (PSO) plane. A standardized preprocedural scan can be used to identify the specific intervertebral space, the estimated US depth to either the epidural space or the subarachnoid space, and, most important, the initial needle insertion site.[26,27] Both the TM and PSO imaging planes can potentially identify the posterior complex (a single linear hyperechoic structure composed of the deepest aspect of the closely adjoining ligamentum flavum, epidural space, and posterior aspect of the dura) and the anterior complex (anterior aspect of the dura, posterior longitudinal ligament, and posterior aspect of the vertebral body) (**Figs. 1** and **2**). The ability to visualize the anterior and/or posterior complex through these open acoustic windows suggests an unobstructed path to the targeted central neuraxial space between either the adjoining spinous processes (via a TM view of the interspinous space) or the adjoining lamina (via a PSO view of the interlaminar space).

Real-Time Ultrasound-Guided Technique

The real-time USG technique requires maintaining the desired imaging plane with one hand while advancing the spinal needle in real time with the other hand. Otherwise, a second operator would be required to either hold the US transducer or advance the needle. This has been described in recent case series[28] but direct comparative studies

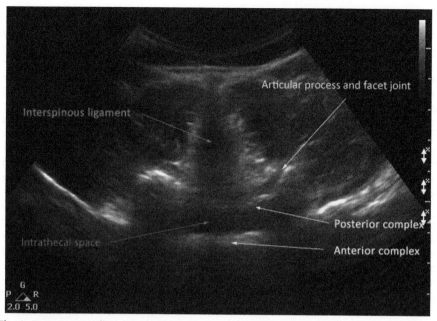

Fig. 1. Transverse midline interlaminar view of the lumbar spine. The interspinous ligament is midline and is located in between adjoining spinous processes. The anterior complex and posterior complex are visible as liner hyperechoic structures, whereas the intrathecal space is the dark hypoechoic area between the anterior and posterior complex.

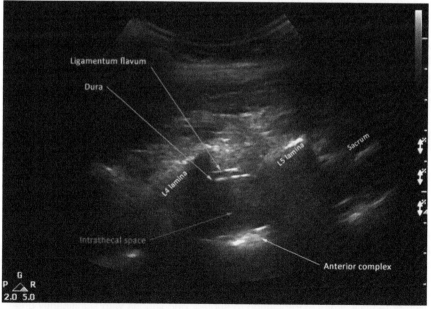

Fig. 2. Paramedian sagittal oblique of the L4-L5 intervertebral space through the interlaminar window. The laminae demonstrate the typical sawtooth appearance. The structures of the spinal canal are visible in between the adjoining lamina. Note the clear visibility of the hyperechoic anterior complex deep to the hypoechoic intrathecal space. Note that the individual components of the posterior complex are clearly visible: the hypoechoic epidural space is located between the ligamentum flavum and posterior aspect of the dura.

to either landmark techniques or preprocedural US-assisted technique are notably lacking.

After the Perlas[8] review, in a quantitative systematic review of central neuraxial analgesia in obstetric subjects (pooled data from three RCTs and three prospective cohort studies in 692 subjects undergoing primarily lumbar epidural analgesia), USG was associated with significant reductions in both needle puncture attempts and fewer punctures levels (sites).[29] More specifically, in subjects in whom it was presumed that central neuraxial blocks would be potentially difficult (obesity, previous lumbar spinal surgery, or a previous history of difficulty), the success rate with USG was 71% compared with only 20% with conventional landmark techniques. That 84% of the data came from a single institution suggests a potential for publication or selection bias (expert or dominating center bias), which limits generalizability of the results.

Since 2010, there have been 5 RCTs that have directly compared US-assisted spinal anesthesia and lumbar epidural analgesia to landmark-based techniques.[30–35] All 5 trials were adequately powered to detect a significant difference in the primary outcomes of interest: successful dural puncture on the first attempt, time required to perform successful block, or success rate of epidural labor analgesia. In all 5 trials, the USG group had a standard preprocedural TM and/or PSO scan to determine the initial needle puncture site, whereas the needle puncture site in the landmark groups was identified by palpation lumbar spinous processes and estimation of the intercristal line.

In the single study investigating labor epidural analgesia in 370 consecutive subjects performed by novice anesthesiology residents, the rate of failed epidural labor analgesia (1.6% vs 5.5%) and insertion attempts (1 vs 2) was significantly lower with USG compared with an landmark-based technique.[30] The preprocedural US scans were performed by a single investigator with substantial experience, raising the possibility that expertise with central neuraxial US may affect success rates when expanded to anesthesiologists with varying degrees of US experience. In an RCT of 150 obstetric spinal anesthetics with easily palpable landmarks in all subjects, USG failed to show a significant difference in procedure time (initial skin puncture to viewing cerebrospinal fluid at the spinal needle hub), number of skin punctures, or needle passes compared with a landmark technique.[31]

In contrast, USG significantly improved the first-pass success rates in a study stratifying subjects as either nonobese (body mass index [BMI] <30 kg/m^2) or obese (>30 BMI kg/m^2).[32] In this study, the first-pass success rate in both nonobese and obese subjects with USG was 92% compared with a first-pass success rate of 72% in nonobese and only 44% in obese subjects without USG. The percentages of difficult or impossible-to-palpate landmarks was similarly high in both the obese US (average BMI = 34.1, 48%) and obese landmark (average BMI = 37.3, 40%) groups, indicating that USG may especially useful when traditional surface anatomic landmarks are difficult to ascertain. Two RCTs have evaluated the usefulness of US-guided spinal anesthesia in nonobstetric subjects.[33,34] In an RCT of 170 subjects scheduled for orthopedic, general surgical, and urologic procedures, USG failed to demonstrate a significant difference in either first-pass success rate or number of needle redirections.[33] In this study, the average BMI in both the US and landmark group was 25, which potentially limits extrapolation to subject populations with significantly greater BMI.

The technical difficulty of spinal anesthesia has been shown to correlate with the quality of palpable surface landmarks.[35,36] In addition to obesity, previous spinal surgery, spinal deformity, or age-related degenerative changes of the lumbar spine may contribute to inaccurate assessment of traditional surface landmarks. An RCT investigated the impact of preprocedural USG on the efficiency of spinal anesthesia in subjects with (1) BMI greater than 35 kg/m², (2) moderate-to-severe lumbar scoliosis, or (3) previous lumbar spinal surgery.[34] In this study, the average BMI (39 vs 41 kg/m²) and percentage of subjects with difficult-to-impossible surface landmarks (61% and 75%) was similarly high in both the US and landmark groups. USG provided an advantage in the primary outcome of first-pass success rate (65% vs 32%), as well decreases in mean number of needle insertion attempts (1 vs 2) and mean number of total needle passes (6 vs 13). The time taken to perform spinal anesthesia was also decreased by an average of 158 seconds with USG. However, the increased time to establish landmarks with USG (6.7 vs 0.6 minutes) compared with landmark-based assessment resulted in the block-related procedure time taking 3.3 minutes longer. Although the block-related time with USG was increased, the decrease in the actual needling time may be more clinically relevant because this is when patients experience discomfort and potential complications may occur.

Although the single RCT looking at a clinically relevant outcome of failed labor epidural analgesia demonstrated an advantage with USG,[30] not unexpectedly, none of the 4 RCTs investigating spinal anesthesia failed to demonstrate an increase in success of surgical anesthesia once cerebrospinal fluid was obtained.[31–34] Additionally, there were no differences in the incidences of unintended paresthesia, nerve, bleeding complications, or postdural puncture headache. All of these patient-related complications are, fortunately, uncommon to rare and it is extremely unlikely that future RCTs will have adequate power to demonstrate an advantage with USG.

USG may also prove useful as screening tool in predicting potentially difficult spinal anesthesia procedures.[37] In a prospective observational study of 60 subjects presenting for lower extremity orthopedic surgery, a standard PSO view of the lumbar spine (see **Fig. 2**) was performed by operators with extensive experience in central neuraxial US. They rated the ability to see the anterior complex and quality of image as either absent, hazy, or clear.[38] Subsequently, another anesthesiologist, blinded to the preprocedural US scan, performed spinal anesthesia. Technically difficult spinal anesthesia was defined as greater than or equal to 10 needle passes and a duration greater than 400 seconds. Poor US visualization of the anterior complex was associated with a 50% rate of difficult spinal anesthesia, whereas the ability to clearly see the anterior complex was associated with only a 9% rate of technical difficulty. More specifically, poor sonographic visualization of the anterior complex was associated with an 82% positive predictive value and a likelihood ratio of 12.8 for difficult spinal anesthesia. In a similar study, experienced operators with central neuraxial US performed preprocedural US in 100 subjects, acquired both TM (see **Fig. 1**) and PSO (see **Fig. 2**) images, and graded images based on the ability to visualize both the anterior and posterior complex.[39] On completion of the US scan, a separate anesthesiologist, blinded to the results of the scan, performed spinal anesthesia guided by conventional landmark techniques via a standard midline approach. Technical difficulty was defined as greater than 2 skin punctures and as greater than 10 needle passes. In this study, although the PSO views provided better image quality of both the anterior and posterior complex than the TM views, only the TM view was accurate in predicting the lack of difficulty with spinal anesthesia (85% positive predictive value). Views obtained in the PSO imaging plane did not have significant diagnostic predictive value for ease of spinal anesthesia via a midline approach. This is not surprising because the PSO imaging plane is directed through the interlaminar space, which is often less narrowed by age-related degenerative changes and typically affords a better acoustic window compared with the TM imaging plane. Thus, it is possible that quality of the PSO view may be a better predictor of technical ease (or difficulty) of spinal anesthesia via paramedian approach; however, this requires further investigation. It is also possible that the image quality obtained with preprocedural TM and PSO views may serve as a guide to using either a midline or paramedian technique needle insertion technique.

REVIEW OF RECENT EVIDENCE FOR ULTRASOUND GUIDANCE AND PATIENT SAFETY

Although data from RCTs and meta-analyses of the pooled data from RCTs provide important data on the efficacy (with high levels of internal validity) of USG versus PNS, conducting an RCT on rare patient-safety outcomes would be cost prohibitive, requiring long study periods and very large numbers of enrolled individuals.[9] Another limitation of RCTs is that they potentially lack external validity (effectiveness or real-world usefulness).[40,41] Data from recently published registries and quality assurance databases have an element of uncertainty in the risk estimate of infrequent events and, due to uncontrolled observational measurements, have a higher risk for unrecognized bias about cause and effect. Nonetheless, they do provide point estimates of risk, especially with infrequently occurring events and, perhaps just as important, reflect real-world clinical practice.[42] Three recently published studies that provide newer data on the incidence of PNI and LAST, with and without USG are summarized.

In a prospective single-center clinical registry[43] of 12,668 USG PNBs over an 8-year period (2003–2011), the reported incidence of long-term PNI was found to be 0.9 (95% CI 0.0–0.3) per 1000 blocks, which is not substantially different than the previously reported 0.4 (95% CI 0.08–1.1) per 1000 blocks from historical controls for both USG and PNS.[9] There was 1 case of LAST (seizure) for a reported incidence of 0.08 (95% CI 0–0.3), highlighting that the incidence is very low. There were no cases of pneumothorax in 1508 USG supraclavicular (SCB) blocks.

In a recent update of a single-center quality assurance database, the incidence of PNI and LAST was reviewed in 9062 PNBs using combined USG with PNS and in 5436 blocks with landmark-based PNS alone.[44] There was no difference in the incidence of long-term PNI between the USG-PNS technique (1 per 9069) and the landmark-PNS technique (7 per 5436). In contrast, there was a statistically-significant difference in the incidence of LAST between US-PNS (0 cases) and landmark-PNS (6 cases). It was notable that the historical incidence of LAST at this single center was 1 to 3 seizures per year (based on 3000–4000 blocks per year) when landmark-PNS was the dominant nerve localization technique. However, over the 6-year study period, the use of USG-PNS increased from approximately 10% to approximately 90%, suggesting that adoption of USG decreased the risk of LAST during this transition period.[12,44]

The most recent update of Australian and New Zealand Registry of Regional Anesthesia (AURORA) further expands the evidence regarding the role of USG in reducing the risk of LAST.[45] The study population of 20,021 subjects who received 25,336 PNBs at 20 hospitals is the largest prospective database to date. There were 22 reported episodes of LAST for an overall incidence of 0.87 (95% CI 0.54–1.3) per 1000 blocks, highlighting that the overall incidence for all PNBs did not differ from previous estimates of LAST.[46] However, there were 10 cases of LAST in the 4745 PNBs without USG for an incidence of 2.1 (95% CI 1.0–3.9) per 1000 blocks. In contrast, there were 12 cases of LAST in 20,401 USG PNBs for an incidence of 0.59 (95% CI 0.30–1.03) per 1000 blocks. The primary finding of this study is that when compared with PNS alone, USG reduced the likelihood of LAST by greater than 65% (odds ratio 0.28, 95% CI 0.12–0.65). However, an accompanying editorial highlighted that USG did not completely eliminate the incidence of LAST[47] and that USG does not eliminate the need for using the minimum effective local anesthetic dose, judicious use of intravascular markers, incremental aspiration and injection, and availability of lipid emulsion and checklists when LAST does occur.[48,49]

Pneumothorax is a potential complication commonly associated with either SCB or ICB approaches to the brachial plexus. The estimated risk of pneumothorax when using non-USG techniques has been reported to be between 0.2% (95% CI 0.0–0.434) and 0.7% (95% CI 0.016–1.318) for ICB[50]; however, it can be as high as 6.1% (95% CI 3–9.2) for SCB.[51] Although a large single-center retrospective analysis did not report a single case of clinically evident pneumothorax with landmark-based SCB in 2020 subjects,[52] the estimated incidence before the USG era had been reported as 0.5% to 6%.[53] There have been no adequately powered RCTs directly comparing USG with landmark-based techniques for either ICB or SCB regarding the risk of pneumothorax.

Recently published large case series do provide updated point estimates of risk. There have been 2 cases of symptomatic pneumothorax in a total of 4736 ICBs,[54–56] with the most recent prospective observational study providing an estimated risk of 0.7% (95% CI 0.0–0.16) or 0.7 per 1000 blocks.[56]

A prospective registry did not report a single case of pneumothorax in 654 USG-SCBs,[57] and in more than 3000 USG-SCBs, a group with substantial experience reported only 1 case of symptomatic pneumothorax over a 4-year period.[58,59] More recently, 2 large prospective observational studies of USG-SCBs have reported an incidence of 0.06 (95% CI 0.0–0.14) in 3403 blocks or 0.6 per 1000 blocks[56] and 0.4 (95% CI 0.01–2.3) in 2384 blocks or 0.4 per 1000 blocks.[60] The reported cases had either immediate or delayed onset of symptoms (typically chest pain and dyspnea) subsequently confirmed by chest radiography. Because routine chest radiography is typically not performed after either ICB or SCB, there is likely a higher incidence of asymptomatic pneumothorax that can spontaneously resolve without sequelae.

EVIDENCE FOR ULTRASOUND GUIDANCE AND CONTINUOUS PERIPHERAL NERVE BLOCKS

CPNBs have been consistently shown to provide superior postoperative pain control and decreased opioid-related side effects compared with both systemic opioid analgesia and single-injection PNBs.[61,62] A recent meta-analysis reviewed 977 subjects in 15 RCTs comparing USG with PNS (both stimulating and nonstimulating catheter techniques). The primary outcome was defined as perioperative successful catheter placement (defined primarily as successful peripheral nerve catheter placement within a defined time period but also included successful surgical block when investigated).[63] Overall, USG provided a modest but statistically significant benefit (relative risk [RR] of 1.14, 95% CI 1.02–1.27) for successful catheter placement with the most benefit occurring with popliteal sciatic and ICB perineural catheter placement, as well as lower risk of accidental vascular puncture (RR 0.13, 95% CI 0.04–0.38). In contrast, postoperative pain scores with movement were comparable between USG versus PNS-guided peripheral nerve catheters. In a unique cost-effectiveness analysis, the incremental cost-effectiveness ratio (ICER; defined as the extra cost per extra successful block) was calculated using 4000 nonparametric bias-corrected bootstrap replicates for USG continuous sciatic nerve block.[64] The mean ICER was negative, indicating that USG leads to better effect and lower cost compared with PNS guidance alone. Subsequent RCTs of CPNBs have focused on comparing 2 primary techniques for USG peripheral perineural catheter placement: short-axis imaging of the target nerve with in-plane (SAX-IP) needle and catheter insertion versus long-axis imaging of the target nerve with in-plane (LAX-IP) needle and catheter insertion; with the primary outcomes investigating either quality of postoperative analgesia or block procedure time.[65–68] Overall, there was no difference in the quality of postoperative analgesia and, not surprisingly, SAX-IP techniques provided a 33% to 45% reduction in the time required for successful catheter placement compared with LAX-IP. Despite the heterogeneity of the study designs within the meta-analyses and RCTs, it seems that USG provides advantages in terms of decreased block procedure time, without advantages in terms of quality of postoperative analgesia. When using USG, the evidence supports that the SAX-IP technique provides advantages in block procedure–related outcomes when compared with alternative approaches.

EVIDENCE FOR OPTIMAL ULTRASOUND-GUIDED LOCAL ANESTHETIC DISTRIBUTION

One of the unique advantages of USG for PNBs is the ability to adjust the needle tip location in real time to optimize local anesthetic distribution either around a nerve or plexus, or within the desired fascial plane or compartment. Although this ability to adjust needle-tip location may potentially offer advantages, multiple needle readjustments may potentially result in increased block procedure time, discomfort, and complications without necessarily increasing block success or block onset time. Several RCTs have been published investigating the optimal LA distribution for successful surgical brachial plexus block and surgical sciatic nerve block.

The most common technique for USG SCB block targets local anesthetic distribution at the intersection of the first rib and subclavian artery in an attempt to anesthetize the inferior trunk (divisions) of the brachial plexus.[69] Described as the *corner pocket technique*, this single-injection technique (SIT) may potentially decrease local anesthetic spread to the more superior aspects of the trunks-divisions. Two RCTs compared SIT *corner pocket technique* (30–35 mL total local anesthetic volume) to a double-injection technique (DIT) (30–35 mL volume equally divided between the corner pocket and the superolateral part of the trunks-divisions) in subjects undergoing surgery of the elbow, forearm, or hand.[70,71] In both studies, DIT provided a more rapid onset of complete sensory block only at 15 minutes (with no difference by 30 minutes) but required more needle passes and longer block procedure time. Thus, there was no difference in anesthesia-related time. More important, the rates of surgical anesthesia were comparable, with the DIT technique offering no clinically significant advantages. In a more recent study comparing SIT (30 mL at the corner pocket) to a triple-injection technique (TIT) for hand, wrist, or elbow surgery. TIT provided a more rapid onset of complete sensory block at 20 minutes but also took longer to perform, with no advantage in rates of successful surgical anesthesia 30 minutes after block completion.[72] For brachial plexus ICB, local anesthetic distribution posterior to the axillary artery (AA) in the sagittal plane appears to be closet to all three 3 cords. RCTs comparing SIT dorsal to the AA to DIT (dorsal and cranial to the AA) or TIT (dorsal, cranial, and inferior to the AA) found no advantages for block onset or block success but longer block procedure times for the multiple-injection techniques.[73,74]

Targeting the 4 terminal nerves of the axillary brachial plexus may potentially provide a more rapid block onset but, intuitively, also requires at least 4 needle passes. A DIT specifically targeting the musculocutaneous nerve in conjunction with circumferential AA local anesthetic spread has been found to be equally efficacious to 4 separate circumferential local anesthetic injections around the musculocutaneous, radial, median, and ulnar nerves (quadruple injection technique) defined as complete block onset and surgical anesthesia by 30 minutes, with fewer needle passes.[75–77] Anatomically, the median nerve is typically located anterior to the AA, whereas the radial nerve is located posterior to the AA.[78] A recent RCT compared DIT (both groups with perineural injections of the musculocutaneous nerve), followed by perivascular (PV) injection either anterior (12 o'clock) or posterior (6 o'clock) to the AA.[79] Interestingly, block performance time, block onset time, and overall block success rate (84%) were comparable in both groups. When cases of block failure were examined, the radial nerve was not blocked in all cases in which local anesthetic PV injection was anterior to the AA, whereas the median nerve was not blocked in all cases in which local anesthetic PV injection was posterior to the artery.

USG for PSNB is an effective and efficient technique for providing surgical anesthesia for major foot and ankle surgery. An USG technique that provides the best balance between rapid and predictable onset of sensory block for surgical anesthesia while minimizing the risk for nerve injury requires an understanding of the complex tissue layers that comprise the popliteal sciatic nerve. The sciatic nerve is formed from 2 nerves: the TN and CPN nerves. They are independent anatomic structures that do not share their respective sensorimotor fibers. The bifurcation (the TN and CPN physically separate) may occur in a range of locations as proximal as the gluteal compartment to as far distal as the popliteal crease; however, it most commonly occurs 5 to 10 cm cephalad to the popliteal crease. Histologically, the sciatic nerve (as with any other peripheral nerve) is composed of both neural tissue (axons) and the surrounding connective tissue.

The non-neural connective tissue has been defined and consists of three layers that have traditionally defined peripheral nerve architecture:[80,81] (1) individual axons are contained within the **endoneurium**; (2) axons are tightly packed within fascicles by the **perineurium** (which serves functionally as the nerve-blood barrier); (3) the **epineurium** comprises all the connective tissue that holds and surrounds the fascicles within the anatomical limit of the peripheral nerve. The epineurium is composed of both an outer (epifascicular) layer and an inner (interfascicular) layer. More recently, anatomic, histologic, and ultrahigh resolution US investigations have defined 2 extraneural connective tissue sheaths[82-84]: (1) the paraneural sheath, composed of multiple circular layers of fascial connective tissue forming an adipose-filled compartment immediately next to and superficial to the epineurium, and (2) an outer epimysial sheath formed from the surrounding muscles, creating a well-defined intermuscular space surrounding the sciatic nerve. The outer 2 connective sheaths form potential compartments for targeted local anesthetic deposition.

Injections deep to the epimysium but external to the paraneural sheath constitute a subepimysial compartment injection and most likely represent the traditional circumferential local anesthetic injection spread (donut sign) that may be achieved above or below the bifurcation of the sciatic nerve.[85-88] Injections deep to the paraneural sheath but external to the epineurium are defined as subparaneural compartment injections. Subparaneural injections can result in both circumferential and longitudinal distribution, thus exposing an extensive surface area of the sciatic nerve to local anesthetic while staying external to the outer boundary of the sciatic nerve.[80,82,84] This summary of the sciatic nerve anatomy provides a background for discussion of a series of RCTs investigating the possible optimal USG local anesthetic distribution for PSNB.

Three RCTs have investigated circumferential subepimysial local anesthetic injections either proximal to the sciatic nerve bifurcation or distal to the sciatic nerve bifurcation. All 3 trials consistently demonstrated a more rapid onset of sensory block with separate subepimysial injections around the smaller TN and CPN components, yet both techniques required multiple needle redirections to achieve circumferential local anesthetic distribution. Two RCTs recently shed light on the potential advantages of injections within the paraneural compartment.[89,90] In these 2 trials, USG was used to direct a needle tip just beyond the bifurcation of the sciatic nerve deep to paraneural sheath, followed by a single injection of local anesthetic. The trials compared block onset time and successful PSNB with the conventional subepimysial circumferential local anesthetic injection around the TN and CPN. Subparaneural injections resulted in significantly more rapid onset of sensory block, increased percentage of complete blocks, and shorter procedure-related block times. Interestingly, subparaneural injections were also associated with more extensive sonographic proximal and longitudinal spread of local anesthetic, without intraneural local anesthetic injection.

SUMMARY

USG has had a profound effect on regional anesthesiology and acute pain medicine. Despite the heterogeneity in the design of multiple RCTs, USG has consistently provided improved outcomes regarding block procedure time, block onset time, and (depending on the varying definitions) increased block success for single-injection and CPNBs. More recent data support a role for preprocedural USG in patients with predictors of technically difficult spinal anesthesia. Although the evidence for decreasing the risk of peripheral injury is currently lacking, accumulating evidence confirms that USG decreases but (just as important) does not eliminate the risk of LAST. Finally, the focus of research has appropriately changed to investigating the optimal USG techniques for specific nerve blocks and emerging data should further expand the applications and benefits of regional anesthesia.

REFERENCES

1. Terkawi AS, Karakitsos D, Elbarbary M, et al. Ultrasound for the anesthesiologist: present and future. ScientificWorldJournal 2013;2013:68365.
2. Matava C, Hayes J. A survey of ultrasound use by academic and community anaesthesiologists in Ontario. Can J Anaesth 2011;58:766–71.
3. Lamperti M, Bodenham AR, Pittiruti M, et al. International evidence-based recommendations on ultrasound-guided vascular access. Intensive Care Med 2012;38:1105–17.
4. Neal JM, Brull R, Chan VW, et al. The ASRA evidence-based medicine assessment of ultrasound-guided regional anesthesia and pain medicine; executive summary. Reg Anesth Pain Med 2010;35:S1–9.
5. McCartney CJ, Lin L, Shastri U. Evidence basis for the use of ultrasound for upper extremity blocks. Reg Anesth Pain Med 2010;35:S10–5.
6. Salinas FV. Ultrasound and review of evidence for lower extremity peripheral nerve blocks. Reg Anesth Pain Med 2010;35:S16–25.
7. Liu SS, Ngeow J, John RS. Evidence basis for ultrasound-guided block characteristics: onset, quality, and duration. Reg Anesth Pain Med 2010;35:S26–35.
8. Perlas A. Evidence for the use of ultrasound in neuraxial blocks. Reg Anesth Pain Med 2010;35:S43–6.
9. Neal JM. Ultrasound-guided regional anesthesia and patient safety: an evidence-based analysis. Reg Anesth Pain Med 2010;35:S59–676.
10. Abrahams MS, Aziz MF, Fu RF, et al. Ultrasound guidance compared with electrical neurostimulation for peripheral nerve block: a systematic review and meta-analysis of randomized controlled trials. Br J Anaesth 2009;102:408–17.
11. Gelfand HJ, Ouanes JPP, Lesley MR, et al. Analgesic efficacy of ultrasound-guided regional anesthesia: a meta-analysis. J Clin Anesth 2011;23:90–6.
12. Laur JJ, Weinberg GL. Comparing safety in surface landmarks versus ultrasound-guided peripheral nerve blocks: an observational study of a practice in transition. Reg Anesth Pain Med 2012;37:569–70.

13. Helwani MA, Saied NN, Asaad B, et al. The current role of ultrasound use in teaching regional anesthesia: a survey of residency programs in the United States. Pain Med 2012;13:1342–6.

14. Sites BD, Neal JM, Chan VW. Ultrasound in regional anesthesia: where should the "focus" be set? Reg Anesth Pain Med 2009;34:531–3.

15. Choquet O, Morau D, Biboulet P, et al. Where should the tip of needle be located in ultrasound-guided peripheral nerve blocks? Curr Opin Anaesthesiol 2012;25:596–602.

16. Sites BD, Chan VW, Neal JM, et al. The American Society of Regional Anesthesia and Pain Medicine and the European Society of Regional Anesthesia and Pain Therapy joint committee recommendations for education and training in ultrasound-guided regional anesthesia. Reg Anesth Pain Med 2012;35:S74–80.

17. Nix CM, Margarido CB, Awad IT, et al. A scoping review of the evidence for teaching ultrasound-guided regional anesthesia. Reg Anesth Pain Med 2013;38:471–80.

18. Thomas LC, Graham SK, Osteen KD, et al. Comparison of ultrasound and nerve stimulation for interscalene brachial plexus block for shoulder surgery in a residency training environment. Oscher J 2011;11:246–53.

19. Cataldo R, Carassiti M, Costa F, et al. Starting with ultrasonography decreases popliteal block performance time in experienced hands; a prospective randomized study. BMC Anesthesiol 2012;12:33.

20. Trabelsi W, Amor MB, Lebbi MA, et al. Ultrasound does not shorten the duration of the procedure, but provides a faster sensory onset and motor block onset in comparison to nerve stimulation in infraclavicular brachial plexus block. Korean J Anesthesiol 2013;64:327–33.

21. Sala-Blanch X, de Riva N, Carrera A, et al. Ultrasound-guided popliteal block with a single injection at the sciatic division results in faster block onset than classical nerve stimulator technique. Anesth Analg 2012;114:1121–7.

22. McNaught A, Shastri U, Carmicheal N, et al. Ultrasound reduces the minimum effective local anaesthetic volume compared with peripheral nerve stimulation for interscalene block. Br J Anaesth 2011;106:124–30.

23. Danelli G, Bonarelli S, Tognu A, et al. Prospective randomized comparison of ultrasound-guided and neurostimulation techniques for continuous interscalene block in patients undergoing coracoacromial ligament repair. Br J Anaesth 2012;108:1006–10.

24. Gautier P, Vandepitte C, Ramquest C, et al. The minimum effective anesthetic volumes of 0.75% ropivacaine in ultrasound-guided brachial plexus block. Anesth Analg 2011;113:951–5.

25. Vandepitte C, Gautier P, Xu D, et al. Effective volume of ropivacaine 0.75% through a catheter required for interscalene brachial plexus block. Anesthesiology 2013;118:863–7.

26. Chin KJ, Karmakar MK, Peng P. Ultrasonography of the adult thoracic and lumbar spine for central neuraxial blockade. Anesthesiology 2011;114:1459–85.

27. Karmakar MK, Li X, Kowk WH, et al. Sonoanatomy relevant for ultrasound-guided central neuraxial blocks via the paramedian approach in the lumbar region. Br J Radiol 2012;85:e262–9.

28. Brinkmann S, Tang R, Sawka A, et al. Single-operator real-time ultrasound-guided spinal injection using SonixGPS™:a case series. Can J Anaesth 2013;69:896–901.

29. Schnabel A, Schuster F, Ermet T, et al. Ultrasound guidance for neuraxial analgesia and anesthesia in obstetrics: a quantitative systematic review. Ultraschall Med 2012;33:E132–7.

30. Vallejo MC, Phelps AL, Singh S, et al. Ultrasound decreases the failed epidural rate in resident trainees. Int J Obstet Anesth 2010;19:373–8.
31. Ansari T, Yousef A, El Gammasy A, et al. Ultrasound-guided spinal anesthesia in obstetrics: is there an advantage over the landmark technique in patients with easily palpable spines. Int J Obstet Anesth 2014;23(3):213–6.
32. Sahin T, Balaban O, Sahin L, et al. A randomized controlled trial of preinsertion ultrasound-guidance for spinal anaesthesia in pregnancy: outcomes among obese and lean parturients: ultrasound for spinal anesthesia in pregnancy. J Anesth 2013;28(3):413–9.
33. Lim YC, Choo CY, Tan TJ. A randomized controlled trial of ultrasound-assisted spinal anesthesia. Anaesth Intensive Care 2014;42:191–8.
34. Chin KJ, Perlas A, Chan VW, et al. Ultrasound imaging facilitates spinal anesthesia in adults with difficult surface anatomical landmarks. Anesthesiology 2011;115:94–101.
35. De Filho GR, Gomes HP, da Fonseca MH, et al. Predictors of successful neuraxial block: a prospective study. Eur J Anaesthesiol 2002;19:447–51.
36. Atallah MM, Demian AD, Shorab AA. Development of difficulty score for spinal anesthesia. Br J Anaesth 2004;92:354–60.
37. Chin KJ, Perlas A. Ultrasonography of the lumbar spine for neuraxial and lumbar plexus blocks. Curr Opin Anaesthesiol 2011;24:567–72.
38. Weed JT, Taenzer AH, Finkel KJ, et al. Evaluation of pre-procedure ultrasound examination as screening tool for difficult spinal anesthesia. Anaesthesia 2011;66:925–30.
39. Chin KJ, Ramlogan R, Arzola C, et al. The utility of ultrasound imaging in predicting ease of performance of spinal anesthesia in an orthopedic patient population. Reg Anesth Pain Med 2013;38:34–8.
40. Memtsoudis SG, Besculides MC. Perioperative comparative effectiveness research. Best Pract Res Clin Anaesthesiol 2011;25:535–47.
41. Kheterpal S. Perioperative comparative effectiveness research; an opportunity calling. Anesthesiology 2009;111:1180–2.
42. Barrington MJ. International registries of regional anesthesia; are we ready to collaborate in virtual departments of anesthesiology? Reg Anesth Pain Med 2012;37:467–9.
43. Sites BD, Taenzer AH, Herrick MD, et al. Incidence of local anesthetic systemic toxicity and postoperative neurological symptoms with 12,668 ultrasound-guided nerve blocks; a prospective clinical registry. Reg Anesth Pain Med 2012;37:478–82.
44. Orebaugh SL, Kentor ML, Williams BD, et al. Adverse outcomes associated with nerve stimulator guided and ultrasound-guided peripheral nerve blocks by supervised trainees; update of a single site database. Reg Anesth Pain Med 2012;37:577–82.
45. Barrington MJ, Kluger R. Ultrasound-guidance reduces the risk of local anesthetic systemic toxicity following peripheral nerve blockade. Reg Anesth Pain Med 2013; 38:289–99.
46. Mulroy MF, Hejtmanek MR. Prevention of local anesthetic systemic toxicity. Reg Anesth Pain Med 2010;35:177–80.
47. Neal JM. Local anesthetic toxicity; improving patient safety one step at a time. Reg Anesth Pain Med 2013;38:259–61.
48. Weinberg GL. Treatment of local anesthetic systemic toxicity. Reg Anesth Pain Med 2010;35:188–93.

49. Neal JM, Mulroy MF, Weinberg GL, et al. American Society of Regional Anesthesia and Pain Medicine checklist for managing local anesthetic systemic toxicity. Reg Anesth Pain Med 2012;37:16–8.
50. Neuberger M, Landes H, Kaiser H. Pneumothorax bei der vertikalen infraklavikularen blockade des plexus brachialis: fallbericht einer seltnenen komplikation. Anaesthesist 2000;49:901–4.
51. Brand L, Papper EM. A comparison of supraclavicular and axillary techniques for brachial plexus block. Anesthesiology 1961;22:253–7.
52. Franco CD, Gloss FJ, Voronov G, et al. Supraclavicular block in obese population: an analysis of 2020 blocks. Anesth Analg 2006;102:1252–4.
53. Brown DL, Bridenbaugh LD. The upper extremity: somatic blockade. In: Cousins MY, Bridenbaugh PO, editors. Neuraxial blockade. 3rd edition. Philadelphia: Lippincott-Raven; 1998. p. 345–70.
54. Sandhu NS, Manne JS, Medebalmi PK, et al. Sonographically guided infraclavicular brachial plexus block in adults: a retrospective analysis of 1146 cases. J Ultrasound Med 2006;25:1555–61.
55. Lecours M, Levesque S, Dion N, et al. Complications of single-injection ultrasound-guided infraclavicular block: a cohort study. Can J Anaesth 2013;60:244–52.
56. Gauss A, Tugtekin I, Georgieff M, et al. Incidence of clinically symptomatic pneumothorax in ultrasound-guided infraclavicular and supraclavicular plexus block. Anaesthesia 2014;69:327–36.
57. Liu SS, Gordon MA, Shaw PS, et al. A prospective clinical registry of ultrasound-guided regional anesthesia for ambulatory shoulder surgery. Anesth Analg 2010;111:617–23.
58. Perlas A, Lobo G, Lo N, et al. Ultrasound-guided supraclavicular block: outcome of 510 consecutive cases. Reg Anesth Pain Med 2009;34:171–6.
59. Brull R, Chan VW. The corner pocket revisited. Reg Anesth Pain Med 2011;36:308.
60. Abell DJ, Barrington MJ. Pneumothorax after ultrasound-guided supraclavicular block: presenting features, risk, and related training. Reg Anesth Pain Med 2014;39:164–7.
61. Richman JM, Liu SS, Courpass G, et al. Does continuous peripheral nerve block provide superior pain control to opioids? A meta-analysis. Anesth Analg 2006; 102:248–57.
62. Bingham AE, Fu R, Horn JL, et al. Continuous peripheral nerve blocks compared with single-injection peripheral nerve blocks; a systematic review and meta-analyses of randomized controlled trials. Reg Anesth Pain Med 2012;37:583–94.
63. Schnabel A, Meyer-Frießern CH, Zahn PK, et al. Ultrasound compared with nerve stimulation guidance for peripheral nerve catheter placement: a meta-analysis of randomized controlled trial. Br J Anaesth 2013;111:564–72.
64. Ehlers L, Jensen JM, Bendtsen TF. Cost-effectiveness of ultrasound vs nerve stimulation guidance for continuous sciatic nerve block. Br J Anaesth 2012; 109:804–8.
65. Wang AZ, Gu LL, Zhou QH, et al. Ultrasound-guided continuous femoral nerve block for analgesia after total knee arthroplasty; catheter perpendicular to the nerve versus catheter parallel to the nerve. Reg Anesth Pain Med 2010;35: 127–31.
66. Mariano ER, Kim TE, Funck N, et al. A randomized comparison of long-and short-axis imaging for in-plane ultrasound-guided femoral perineural catheter insertion. J Ultrasound Med 2013;32:149–56.

67. Fredrickson MI, Danesh-Clough TK. Ultrasound-guided femoral catheter placement: a randomized comparison of in-plane and out-of-plane techniques. Anaesthesia 2013;68:382–90.

68. Kim TE, Howard SK, Funck N, et al. A randomized comparison of long-axis and short-axis imaging for in-plane ultrasound-guided popliteal sciatic perineural catheter insertion. J Anesth 2014;33:1653–62.

69. Soares LG, Brull R, Lai J, et al. Eight-ball, corner pocket: the optimal needle position for ultrasound-guided supraclavicular block. Reg Anesth Pain Med 2007;32:94–5.

70. Tran de QH, Munoz L, Zaouter C, et al. A prospective, randomized comparison between single-and-double-injection, ultrasound-guided supraclavicular block. Reg Anesth Pain Med 2009;34:420–4.

71. Roy M, Nadeau MJ, Cote D, et al. Comparison of single-or double-injection technique for ultrasound-guided supraclavicular block: a prospective randomized, blinded controlled study. Reg Anesth Pain Med 2011;37:55–9.

72. Desgagnes MC, Levesque S, Dion N, et al. A comparison of single or triple injection technique for ultrasound-guided infraclavicular block: a prospective randomized controlled study. Anesth Analg 2009;109:668–72.

73. Fredrickson MJ, Wolstencroft P, Kejriwal R, et al. Single versus triple injection ultrasound-guided infraclavicular block: confirmation of the effectiveness of the single injection technique. Anesth Analg 2010;111:1325–7.

74. Tran de QH, Bertini P, Zaouter C, et al. A prospective, randomized comparison between single-injection and double-injection ultrasound-guided infraclavicular brachial plexus block. Reg Anesth Pain Med 2001;35:16–21.

75. Imasogie N, Ganapathy S, Singh S, et al. A prospective, randomized, double-blind comparison of using ultrasound-guided axillary brachial plexus blocks using 2 versus 4 injections. Anesth Analg 2010;110:1222–6.

76. Tran de QH, Pham K, Dugani S, et al. A prospective randomized comparison between double-, triple-, and quadruple-injection ultrasound-guided axially brachial plexus block. Reg Anesth Pain Med 2012;37:248–53.

77. Bernucci F, Gonzalez AP, Finlayson RJ, et al. A prospective, randomized, comparison between perivascular and perineural ultrasound-guided axillary brachial plexus block. Reg Anesth Pain Med 2012;37:473–7.

78. Christophe JL, Berthier F, Boillot A, et al. Assessment of topographical brachial plexus nerves variations at the axilla using ultrasonography. Br J Anaesth 2009; 103:606–12.

79. Cho S, Kim YJ, Kim JH, et al. Double-injection perivascular block according to needle position: 12 versus 6 o'clock position of the axillary artery. Korean J Anesthesiol 2014;66:112–9.

80. Franco CD. Connective tissue associated with peripheral nerves. Reg Anesth Pain Med 2012;37:363–5.

81. Reina MA, Arriazu R, Collier CB, et al. Electron microscopy of human peripheral nerves of clinical relevance to the practice of peripheral nerve blocks: a structural and ultrastructural review based on original experimental and laboratory data. Rev Esp Anestesiol Reanim 2013;60:552–652.

82. Andersen HL, Andersen SL, Tranum-Jensen J, et al. Injection inside the paraneural sheath of the sciatic nerve: direct comparison among ultrasound imaging, macroscopic anatomy, and histological analysis. Reg Anesth Pain Med 2012; 37:410–4.

83. Karmakar MK, Shariat AN, Panthipampai P, et al. High-definition ultrasound defines the paraneural sheath and fascial compartments surrounding the sciatic nerve at the popliteal fossa. Reg Anesth Pain Med 2013;38:447–51.

84. Abdallah FW, Chan VW. The paraneural compartment: a new destination? Reg Anesth Pain Med 2013;38:375–7.
85. Brull R, Macfarlane AJ, Parrington SJ, et al. Is circumferential injection advantageous for ultrasound-guided popliteal sciatic nerve block? A proof of concept study. Reg Anesth Pain Med 2011;36:266–70.
86. Prasad A, Perlas A, Ramlogan R, et al. Ultrasound-guided popliteal block distal to the sciatic nerve bifurcation shortens onset time: a prospective randomized double-blind study. Reg Anesth Pain Med 2010;35:267–71.
87. Germain G, Lévesque S, Dion N, et al. A comparison of injection cephalad or caudad to the division of the sciatic nerve for ultrasound-guided popliteal: a prospective randomized study. Anesth Analg 2012;114:233–5.
88. Buys MJ, Ardnt CD, Vagh F, et al. Ultrasound-guided sciatic nerve block in the popliteal fossa using a lateral approach: onset time comparing separate tibial and common peroneal injections versus proximal to the bifurcation. Anesth Analg 2010;110:635–7.
89. Tran De QH, Dugani S, Pham K, et al. A randomized comparison between subepineural and conventional ultrasound-guided popliteal sciatic nerve block. Reg Anesth Pain Med 2011;36(6):548–52.
90. Perlas A, Wong P, Abdallah F, et al. Ultrasound-guided popliteal block through a common paraneural sheath versus conventional injection; a prospective, randomized, double-blind study. Reg Anesth Pain Med 2013;38:218–25.

Role of Regional Anesthesia in Orthopedic Trauma

Laura Clark, MD*, Marjorie Robinson, MD, Marina Varbanova, MD

KEYWORDS

- Regional anesthesia • Orthopedic trauma • Risks and benefits of regional anesthesia
- Regional anesthesia techniques • Battlefield anesthesia

KEY POINTS

- In the past and more recently, regional anesthesia has played a central role in the treatment of patients with orthopedic trauma in the battlefield.
- Benefits of regional anesthesia include reduced morbidity and mortality, decreased reliance on opioids with improved postoperative pain management, decreased incidence of deep venous thrombosis, potential reduction in the development of chronic pain, improved participation in rehabilitation, and shorter hospital stays.
- Regional analgesia is a complement to an overall multimodal acute pain therapy and is, therefore, a therapeutic intervention that improves the outcome of the patient with trauma rather than an adjunct to provide pain relief.
- Neuraxial and peripheral nerve block techniques can be safely used in patients with orthopedic trauma and are selected based on the location of the injury.
- When performing regional anesthesia for patients with trauma, coexisting injures, positioning, coagulation status, risk of compartment syndrome, infection, nerve injury, and sedation status must all be taken into consideration.

INTRODUCTION
Trauma and the Role of the Anesthesiologist

Trauma continues to be a major cause of morbidity and mortality worldwide. In the United States, trauma is the number 1 cause of death in patients between the ages of 1 and 44 years and the number 3 cause of death overall. Trauma is responsible for 180,000 deaths, 41 million emergency room visits, and 2 million hospital

Funding Sources: None.
Conflicts of Interest: None.
Department of Anesthesiology and Perioperative Medicine, University of Louisville School of Medicine, 530 S Jackson Street, C2A01, Louisville, KY 40202, USA
* Corresponding author.
E-mail address: mickai@aol.com

admissions each year. The toll of trauma on the health care system and health care spending is significant, with the economic burden of trauma more than $406 billion annually.[1]

Patients with trauma present a unique challenge to the anesthesiologist. On presentation, stabilization of the patient remains the primary concern with focus on cardiopulmonary resuscitation, hemodynamics, and multifocal injuries that may lead to end-organ damage. The medical history and full extent of the patient's injuries are often unknown during this phase. In this environment, managing the patient's pain is a complex but crucial task. Inadequate pain management can have deleterious consequences both in the acute postinjury period and in the long term with increases in chronic pain syndromes. The evidence of the inadequacy of morphine as a sole treatment of pain has recently expanded and the treatment of pain based on morphine as the primary agent has undergone extensive revision. Opioid-induced depression of the immune system, increased reporting of complications caused by morphine, and the development of new drugs such as intravenous agents and local anesthetic preparations has ushered in a more comprehensive treatment modality in which regional anesthetic plays an important complementary role. The anesthesiologist is on the forefront to initiate and coordinate the use of multimodal analgesia and regional analgesia to maximize pain control in these complex patients. Multimodal analgesia involves the use of an array of pharmacologic agents, each with unique mechanisms, to treat pain. These agents include opioids, nonsteroidal antiinflammatory drugs, alpha-2 agonists, N-methyl-D-aspartate antagonists, anticonvulsants, and antidepressants. Regional anesthesia, as a component of multimodal analgesia, is paramount in the trauma population as a means of controlling pain with few to no systemic side effects. Both neuraxial and peripheral nerve block techniques can be used in patients with orthopedic trauma, therefore anesthesiologists must be well trained in both techniques for controlling pain from various injuries. They must also take into account the coagulation status of the patient, as well as the possibility of compartment syndrome, peripheral nerve injury, and infection. With these considerations in mind, regional anesthesia can play a central role in the pain management of each patient with trauma.

History of Pain Relief for Patients with Orthopedic Trauma and the Role of Regional Anesthesia in the Battlefield

Orthopedic trauma has been a major cause of morbidity throughout human history, and attempts to manage pain caused by trauma can be dated back to early civilizations. The first use of opium, like the preparations for analgesia, was recorded in 1500 BC. The compressing of peripheral nerves, for extended periods of time, to cause analgesia distal to the site of compression is a historical method of regional anesthesia described in the sixteenth century by Ambroise Paré, a French military surgeon. The first effective local anesthetic, cocaine, was isolated in 1859. In the years following this discovery, most of the regional anesthesia techniques were developed that continue to be used today.[2] Conduction anesthesia was discovered by William Halstead (1852–1922); Harvey Cushing introduced the term regional anesthesia in 1901; and the Bier block was introduced in 1908, in which Bier[3] described the intravenous injection of local anesthetics. Ansbro's[4] performance of the first continuous nerve block occurred in 1946, and the first epidural anesthesia performance was by Corning[5] in 1885. The clinical history of spinal anesthesia can be dated back to August Bier and August Hildebrandt in 1899.[6]

In the past, the treatment of traumatic pain in civilians also benefited from advancements made in medicine on the battlefield. The optimization of pain management originating from battlefield trauma stretches across many disciplines. However, not until recent military experiences has the concept of acute pain, as a pathophysiologic process with the potential to develop into the disease process of chronic pain, come to the forefront.[7] Pain management in wounded soldiers from the Iraq and Afghanistan wars has improved significantly compared with previous military conflicts. This improvement can be attributed to the introduction of continuous peripheral nerve block (CPNB) techniques and advances of medical delivery technologies.[8] Soldiers returning from recent conflicts have also had a high incidence of polytraumatic injuries with a significant percentage requiring numerous orthopedic interventions.[8,9] At present, few studies show the impact of early aggressive analgesia with acute pain service involvement at combat support hospitals. Buckenmaier and colleagues[10] showed a statistically significant decrease in pain intensity and an increase in pain relief in 71 soldiers sustaining major combat injury treated with aggressive multimodal analgesia interventions including regional nerve blocks.

In a survey completed after being evacuated from Iraq and Afghanistan between July 2007 and February 2008, 110 wounded soldiers reported that average pain relief was 45.2% ± 26.6% during transport and 64.5% ± 23.5% while at the at Landstuhl Regional Medical Center (LRMC) in Germany. Participants with CPNB catheters, placed at LRMC, reported significantly less pain and better pain relief than soldiers without regional anesthesia.[11]

Neurochemistry of Nociception in Trauma

Nociception is the process of biochemical and neural change in response to painful stimuli. It includes the transduction, transmission, modulation, and perception of pain. Transduction is the conversion of tissue injury and a biochemical response to a neural response. The inflammatory mediators implicated in pain and hyperalgesia include bradykinins, potassium, cytokines, substance P, histamine, serotonin, prostacyclin, leukotrienes, and prostaglandins.

Following trauma, injured tissues release local inflammatory mediators causing vasodilation, erythema, and swelling in the affected area. Injury also activates distinct peripheral nociceptors. Peripheral nociceptors are nerves (C fibers and A fibers) that transmit the pain signal along the axon of the primary afferent neuron to their cell bodies in the dorsal root ganglia. After reaching the root ganglia the signal is directed centrally by synapsing onto secondary neurons in the dorsal horn of the spinal cord. In order for the nociceptive stimulus to be interpreted as pain, the nociceptive information must be transmitted from the periphery to the cerebral cortex. This process is accomplished in this order:

- Primary sensory neurons (afferents) conduct the nociceptive information from the periphery to the spinal cord (dorsal horn) and the central nervous system.
- Nociceptive information is transmitted from the spinal cord to the thalamus by the anterolateral system (spinothalamic tract) and the dorsal column medial lemniscal system.
- From the thalamus, nociceptive information can be transmitted to the cerebral cortex resulting in subsequent response(s) to the noxious stimulus.[12]

More complex pathways contribute to the intensity of pain. Thus, there are 3 sites (periphery, spinal cord, and brain) available for modulation by the different modalities of pain control. The periphery and spinal cord are the primary targets for regional anesthesia techniques in orthopedic trauma. Traumatized tissue releases algesic agents that excite the primary afferent fibers and stimulate the hypothalamic-pituitary-adrenal axis. The hormones released because of this stress response to trauma include corticotropin-releasing hormone, adrenocorticotropic hormone, beta-endorphins, epinephrine, norepinephrine, cortisol, antidiuretic hormone, vasopressin, aldosterone, glucagon, and growth hormone. As a result of the release of these hormones, several effects occur in the patient: hypertension, tachycardia, increased oxygen consumption, increased catabolism, a hypercoagulable state, immune system suppression, decreased anabolism, and water and salt retention.

The ebb phase following acute trauma typically lasts 24 hours. This phase is characterized by receptor-mediated vasoconstriction, decreased urine flow, decreased oxygen use, and increased stress hormone levels. The ebb phase is followed by the flow phase, which typically lasts between 2 and 5 days. It involves an increase of cardiac output, increase of oxygen consumption, increase in beta-adrenoreceptor mediation in regional blood flow, and a hypermetabolic state.[12] The hypermetabolic response to trauma results in several changes: increased lipolysis and ketogenesis, increased muscle proteolysis, increased gluconeogenesis and glycogenolysis, insulin resistance, and increased lactate production in skeletal muscle. The primary injury phase in the posttrauma response is followed by an inflammatory phase. This inflammatory phase is associated with the release of traditional inflammatory mediators such as cytokines, leukotrienes, neuropeptides, nitric oxide, and nerve growth factor. This "inflammatory soup" may cause sensitization of nociceptors as well as providing persistent input to the spinal cord, which contributes to the pain pattern in the post-injury phase even after the stimulus has receded.[12]

Benefits of Regional Anesthesia and Analgesia in Orthopedic Trauma

Uncontrolled pain may contribute to morbidity through activation of a stress response and the coagulation cascade. This process results in an increased activity of the sympathetic nervous system, which causes increased myocardial oxygen demand because of increased heart rate, contractility, and systemic vascular resistance. In addition, it can enhance hypercoagulability, which contributes to vasospasm and thrombosis, which is especially undesirable in patients with trauma. Experimental data suggest that thoracic epidural anesthesia with local anesthetics can reduce sympathetic activation and provide a favorable balance of oxygen supply and demand to the myocardium.[13] The relief of pain with neuraxial or peripheral nerve block, when indicated, can be a key in a successful management of patients with orthopedic trauma.

Advantages of Regional Anesthesia in Orthopedic Trauma

- Improved postoperative pain management and decreased incidence of delirium
- Ability to evaluate mental status changes
- Decreased incidence of deep venous thrombosis
- Improved vascular flow
- Decreased blood loss
- Reduced morbidity and mortality
- Facilitation of early mobilization
- Shorter overall hospital stay in orthopedic patients receiving peripheral nerve blocks[4]

The beneficial effect of regional anesthesia in orthopedic trauma is the modulation of pain and the subsequent sympathetic response. In addition, a sympathetic blockade (specifically with neuraxial anesthesia and local anesthetics) allows parasympathetic (vagal) activity to dominate. It is generally thought that the vagal afferent nerve pathway dominates the response to mild and moderate peripheral inflammation, whereas strong inflammatory signals are transmitted to the brain through hormonal mechanisms.[14] The vagus nerve controls and modulates the peripheral inflammatory status by signaling directly to macrophages and microvascular endothelial cells.[15] Other advantages of regional anesthesia in orthopedic trauma include the ability to assess mental status, improved postoperative pain management, decreased blood loss and incidence of venous thrombosis, increased vascular flow, avoidance of airway instrumentation, and facilitation of physical therapy and early mobilization.[16] In a recently published study[17] using a large nationwide sample, use of neuraxial anesthesia was associated with better perioperative outcomes after primary hip and knee arthroplasty compared with general anesthesia. This finding suggests that neuraxial anesthesia represents a positive modifier in reducing perioperative complications and that the type of anesthesia used might have a larger impact on orthopedic patient outcomes than previously assumed.

Improved Outcomes in Patients Receiving Neuraxial Anesthesia Compared with General Anesthesia

- Eighty percent lower 30-day mortality
- Thirty percent lower risk of prolonged length of hospital stay and increased patient cost
- Between 30% and 50% lower risk of major complications including stroke, pneumonia, kidney failure, and the need for mechanical ventilation.

PERIOPERATIVE REGIONAL TECHNIQUES IN ORTHOPEDIC TRAUMA
Neuraxial Techniques

Spinal and epidural analgesia are often not indicated for the primary operation except in isolated injuries such as a hip or acetabular fracture because of hemodynamic instability in patients with trauma and the possibility of unknown injuries. However, continuous epidural or paravertebral analgesia is routinely used as a means of postoperative analgesia in patients with trauma with rib fractures or primary abdominal injuries. It may improve patient morbidity by decreasing pulmonary, cardiovascular, and gastrointestinal complications.[18] Perioperative epidural infusion can be delivered as a fixed continuous infusion, patient-controlled epidural analgesia (PCEA), or most frequently the combination of a basal continuous infusion with PCEA. Clinicians must consider the following contraindications to neuraxial anesthesia:

- Patient refusal or inability to cooperate
- Sepsis or local infection at needle insertion site
- Severe hypervolemia or hemodynamic instability
- Coagulation disorders or anticoagulation therapy
- Increased intracranial pressure

In addition, there are considerations specific to patients with trauma. Positioning may be difficult in patients with multifocal or spine injuries. The spine must be radiographically clear and imaging studies reviewed before placing a catheter. The location of epidural placement is dictated by the site of injury and desired analgesia. Thoracic epidurals are recommended for chest and abdominal trauma, including rib fractures. Lumbar epidurals are used to for trauma and orthopedic procedures involving the lower extremities.

Paravertebral Block

The paravertebral block has an important place in the armamentarium of the anesthesiologist who treats patients with orthopedic trauma. This block involves injecting local anesthetic close to the vertebra at the level where the spinal nerves exit the intervertebral foramina. An ipsilateral somatic and sympathetic block is achieved that extends longitudinally above and below the injected vertebral level. This block may be ipsilateral or bilateral and may be performed as single-shot injection of 15 to 20 mL of local anesthetic or with the placement of a paravertebral catheter. A paravertebral block has been shown to provide pain relief equal to that provided by an epidural after multiple rib fractures. In our experience of large extensive rib fractures, an epidural may be preferred to 2 to 4 paravertebral catheters to cover the extensive injuries. A case series by Karmakar and colleagues,[19] the advantages of thoracic paravertebral block included improved respiratory parameters and oxygenation.

Peripheral Nerve Blocks

Peripheral nerve blocks of both the upper and lower extremity can be performed for treatment of pain in these areas. The specific nerve block used is based on the site of injury and the planned operative procedure. As with neuraxial blockade, there are contraindications to peripheral nerve blocks. These contraindications are relative and the risk and benefit of the block should be considered for the individual patient. Relative contraindications include the following:

- Uncooperative patient
- Bleeding diathesis
- Infection at the site of injection or evidence of bacteremia
- Local anesthetic toxicity (when using multiple site analgesic technique clinicians must take into consideration the total amount of local anesthetic infused)
- Peripheral neuropathy (such as contralateral phrenic nerve palsy)[20]

Upper extremity nerve blocks

For injuries involving the shoulder, a brachial plexus block at the interscalene or supra-clavicular location is used. For more distal injures involving the upper and lower arm and the hand, the supraclavicular, infraclavicular, and axillary approaches to the brachial plexus are used. Because patients with trauma are often in a cervical collar, investigation into the underlying cervical injury is necessary. In situations in which cervical imaging is negative, the C-collar may be removed and the head stabilized to allow placement of the block. In addition, a high supraclavicular block may be used in place of an interscalene approach in situations that necessitate avoidance of head or neck movement. The infraclavicular approach for analgesia of the upper extremity from the elbow to the hand is ideal in patients with trauma because it involves no movement of the head and neck. The axillary approach is perhaps the least desirable in patients with trauma because it requires movement of the injured extremity. Specific consideration unique to patients with trauma must be taken into account when placing upper extremity nerve blocks. The interscalene approach causes hemidiaphragmatic paresis with a 25% to 30% reduction in pulmonary function[21] and thus is not preferable in patients with poor respiratory reserve or contralateral pneumothorax. Although the incidence of hemidiaphragmatic paresis is less in patients undergoing a supraclavic-ular approach, caution should be exercised in patients with underlying pulmonary compromise. The supraclavicular and infraclavicular approaches also have the risk of pneumothorax. In addition, during approaches above the clavicle and infraclavic-ular approach, the local anesthetic can spread to the cervical sympathetic chain causing Horner syndrome or result in anesthesia of the recurrent laryngeal nerve causing hoarseness or difficulty swallowing.

The presence of traumatic nerve injury is not a contraindication for an upper extrem-ity block. However, there must be a discussion with the surgeon, and the surgeon must agree to the plan. The nerve injury must be documented before the block, which in some instances includes a drawing.

If evaluation of the nerve is desired soon after surgery a short-acting local anesthetic can be used and the analgesia restarted after the evaluation.

Lower extremity nerve blocks

All peripheral nerve blocks effective for the lower extremity may be performed for analgesia of pain from traumatic injury. The sciatic nerve may be blocked from the level of the sacral plexus to the popliteal fossa by multiple approaches including anterior, posterior, and lateral. The choice of approach depends on the location of the injury, the operative procedure, and the ability to position the patient. Lumbar plexus blocks can provide analgesia for the hip, femoral neck, and shaft, as well as the knee joint. They are also useful for pain management after open reduction and internal fixation of acetabular fractures. Chelly and colleagues[22] placed a series of 13 lumbar plexus catheters postoperatively in anesthetized patients who had undergone open reduction and internal fixation of acetabular fractures. A continuous infusion reduced morphine requirements by nearly 60%. Femoral nerve blocks and fascia iliaca compartment blocks are both used for analgesia in patients with femoral neck fractures. Newman and colleagues[23] conducted a randomized controlled trial of 110 patients to compare the analgesic efficacy and opioid-sparing effect of the two techniques. They found superior efficacy and reduced consumption of morphine with the femoral nerve block. The combination of a femoral or saphenous block (or catheter) with sciatic block (or catheter) can provide excellent analgesia for the entire lower extremity.

Single-injection blocks versus continuous catheter techniques

Peripheral nerve blocks may be performed as a single injection or by placement of a CPNB catheter. The decision should be based primarily on the extent and duration of severe pain from the injury and/or surgery. Many traumatic injuries are not candidates for a single-shot block, because the pain is likely to be present for 24 hours to several days. Single-injection nerve blocks can provide analgesia for a period of only 10 to 24 hours even with long-acting local anesthetics such as bupivacaine and ropivacaine. Single-injection nerve blocks may be preferable in patients in whom potential infection of an indwelling catheter is a concern. However, Buckenmaier and colleagues[24] and others showed that infection in continuous catheters was rare in the battlefield.[25] Lai and colleagues[26] studied 6 case reports and found that risk factors include duration of catheter placement, type of catheter, preprocedural antibiotics, and tunneled versus nontunneled catheters. CPNBs allow prolonged delivery of local anesthetic to the site that requires analgesia. This ability is especially important in patients with orthopedic trauma, who often have postoperative or posttraumatic extremity pain that persists beyond 24 hours. The patency of catheters is usually 2 to 3 days, but can be 1 to 2 weeks or, in rare instances, even longer. Often the logistics of taking care of the patient with a catheter, as well as the increased time for placement, has been a determent to their use. This practice does not take into consideration the merits and the unique advantages of continuous analgesia. The analgesic advantages of CPNBs mean that they need to be recategorized as a therapeutic intervention rather than an optional accessory when convenient. The implementation of an acute pain service can alleviate those determents. Recent data show that the use of ultrasonography can decrease the time needed to place perineural catheters compared with the time required using traditional nerve stimulation techniques.[27,28]

The simultaneous use of multiple continuous nerve block catheters in the same patient is common in cases of multiple orthopedic traumas. The concerns of multiplying the risks in this group seem logical, but there are no publications reporting increased toxicity or increased infection rate linked to having multiple catheters at the same time in 1 patient.

The safety of long-term infusion of ropivacaine in peripheral nerve catheters was recently investigated in a study by Bleckner and colleagues.[29] Free serum ropivacaine concentrations in 35 patients with trauma with peripheral nerve catheters infused with ropivacaine 0.2% or as a bolus with ropivacaine 0.5% were measured at time points of 3, 5, 7, and 10 days and then every third day until catheter removal. Continuous ropivacaine infusion over a prolonged period did not produce toxic or near-toxic serum concentrations.

The current authors reported a case of a 37-year-old female patient with polytrauma who benefited greatly from the placement of CPNB catheters that were maintained over multiple surgeries. The patient sustained multiple injuries when her home collapsed on her during a tornado. These injuries included extensive soft tissue and degloving injuries to bilateral lower extremities and multiple rib fractures. Following initial bilateral amputations, right below-knee amputation and left above-knee amputation, bilateral femoral catheters and bilateral sciatic catheters were placed. The femoral catheters were placed under ultrasonography guidance. The sciatic catheters, 1 gluteal and 1 subgluteal, were placed with nerve stimulation because excessive edema prevented ultrasonography identification of the sciatic nerve. Ropivacaine 0.2% was infused at 7 mL/h via the bilateral femoral catheters and at 4 mL/h via the bilateral sciatic catheters for 14 days. Sensory block was achieved with motor function remaining intact. During her hospital admission period of 14 days, she underwent additional surgical procedures including washouts, revisions, and a closure procedure throughout which the catheters remained in place. The patient had excellent pain control and no reports of phantom sensation or phantom limb pain. The patient discontinued opioid pain medications less than 1 week after hospital discharge. Following rehabilitation, she was able to ambulate well with bilateral lower extremity prostheses. This case example shows the benefit of early aggressive pain treatment and the utility of prolonged peripheral nerve catheters for sustained pain relief in patients with orthopedic trauma.

There has also been investigation into the role of continuous peripheral nerve catheters in the outpatient setting. In many institutions, orthopedic surgery outpatients are discharged home with a continuous peripheral nerve catheter infusion of local anesthetic that they remove within a few days following surgery. Ilfeld and colleagues[30] investigated the use of CPNB infusion in a pilot study of 3 patients with a chronic condition of intractable phantom limb pain following amputation. Favorable results in these few patients suggest that this may be a beneficial treatment in the amputee population.

The difference in catheter types, insertion techniques, and a variety of other factors makes the recommendation of optimal infusion rate in patients with multiple catheters difficult. Most published investigations report a basal rate of 4 to 10 mL/h (lower rates for catheters of the lower extremities; higher rates for the upper extremity), a bolus of 2 to 10 mL, and a bolus lockout period of 20 to 60 minutes. The maximum hourly rate of total dose of local anesthetic during perineural infusion remains unknown. One study reported no toxicity signs or symptoms with perineural ropivacaine 0.2% administered at basal rates up to 14 mL/h and large repeated boluses of ropivacaine 0.5% (10–60 mL) provided up to 27 days.[31] A case report of a patient with trauma exposed to an improvised explosive device noted the simultaneous use of infraclavicular continuous catheter (infusing ropivacaine at 10 mL/h with 3-mL bolus every 20 minutes), bilateral sciatic catheters, and 1 femoral catheter with infusions at 10 mL/h each, in addition to 5 mL every 30 minutes demand dose in each sciatic catheter. The patient's serum ropivacaine levels were analyzed 24 hours after the start of the infusions and were 5.8 mg/L and less than 0.1 mg/L for total and free concentrations, respectively.[32]

Regional Analgesia for Crush Injuries

CPNBs benefit a subset of patients with orthopedic trauma who have sustained a crush injury to an extremity with concomitant disrupted blood flow. The sympathetic nerves are closely related to the blood vessels in the neurovascular bundle. Therefore peripheral nerve blockade with attendant sympathetic block is used to induce vasodilation and increase blood flow after a vascular injury. One early report describes the successful use of a continuous brachial plexus block in a series of 3 patients with upper extremity vascular injuries.[33] Another article documented improved circulation and healing with continuous blockade following microvascular digit transfer and reimplantation surgery.[34] A more recent report describes the use of a continuous brachial plexus catheter for sympathectomy and distal limb perfusion in a child following near amputation and extensive reconstructive surgery.[35]

Suggested regional anesthetic techniques for specific orthopedic injuries are shown in **Table 1**.

LOCAL ANESTHETICS AND ANALGESIC ADJUVANTS FOR REGIONAL ANESTHESIA
Neuraxial Blocks

Local anesthetics are the most commonly used medications for neuraxial analgesia. Their principal mechanism of action is the arrest of nerve conduction by blocking sodium channels. Central neuraxial blockade occurs at the level of the spinal nerve root. Local anesthetic solutions alone can provide excellent analgesia but may produce concomitant sympathetic and motor blockade, which can cause side effects of hypotension from sympathetic blockade and limitation of ambulation from motor blockade. Opioids are another pharmacologic agent commonly used in epidural infusions for analgesia. Opioid penetration into the spinal cord is both time and concentration dependent. The lipophilicity of the particular opioid also plays a role in the analgesic profile. For example, hydrophilic agents such as morphine produce analgesia at lower blood levels than lipophilic agents such as fentanyl. Epidural opioids alone may produce significant dose-dependent side effects. The most serious of these is respiratory depression resulting from the diffusion of the opioid into the cerebrospinal fluid and migration to the medullary respiratory center. Other side effects of epidural opioids

Table 1
Suggested regional anesthetic techniques for specific orthopedic injuries

Injury Location	Suggested Regional Anesthetic Technique
Rib	Thoracic epidural or paravertebral block
Pelvis	Epidural
Femoral neck	Lumbar plexus, femoral, or fascia iliaca
Femoral shaft	Femoral
Knee	Femoral, sciatic
Patella	Femoral
Ankle	Femoral, sciatic
Foot	Sciatic
Shoulder	Interscalene, supraclavicular
Upper/lower arm or hand	Supraclavicular, infraclavicular axillary

include itching, nausea, urinary retention, sedation, and ileus. Therefore dilute local anesthetic infusions are often combined with opioids to achieve optimal analgesia with low incidence of side effects. The authors currently use an infusion of ropivacaine 0.1% with fentanyl 5 μg/mL or ropivacaine 0.1% with hydromorphone 10 μg/mL at a basal infusion rate of 5 to 10 mL/h with an additional PCEA dose.

Peripheral Nerve Blocks

Local anesthetics are the principal agents in peripheral nerve blocks. In selecting an agent, the anesthesiologist must consider the characteristics of the agents:

- Time to onset
- Duration of action
- Degree of sensory versus motor block
- Cardiac toxicity

Bupivacaine offers the advantages of long duration and sensory blockade compared with motor blockade. However, it has a potential for cardiac toxicity, including cardiac arrhythmias and arrest. Ropivacaine offers the same duration profile with less potential for cardiac side effects. Ropivacaine solutions of 0.1% to 0.2% seem to offer the best range for balancing sensory and motor blockade during continuous infusion. One study of popliteal sciatic blocks found that a concentrated solution in smaller volume seems preferable.[36] Other adjunct pharmacologic agents have been studied in peripheral nerve blocks. These agents include epinephrine, clonidine, dexmedetomidine, buprenorphine, dexamethasone, sodium bicarbonate, tramadol, and midazolam. Epinephrine is the most widely used adjunct for peripheral nerve blockade. Experts agree that the use of epinephrine may increase potential neurotoxicity, especially in high-risk patients. They recommend the use of epinephrine only for nerve blocks done without ultrasonography guidance or blocks in which needle tip and local anesthetic spread is not adequately visualized as a safety measure against intravascular injection.[37] Clonidine, an alpha-2 agonist, has been added to the local anesthetic; multiple reviews and meta-analyses show both an analgesic benefit and side effects. The sedation and hypotension possibility and lack of duration beyond the local anesthetic has limited its use, especially in patients with trauma. The use of a newer alpha-2 agonist, dexmedetomidine, has also been used to a more limited extent as an additive. A recent study in which dexmedetomidine was added to levobupivacaine for axillary nerve blocks showed improved onset time and increased duration of anesthesia.[38] Although the use of traditional opioids has not been shown to be effective in peripheral nerve blocks, buprenorphine, a mu agonist and kappa antagonist, was shown to give an analgesic advantage to local anesthetic.[39] The addition of dexamethasone, as described in 2 recent publications, is gaining popularity in perineural local anesthetic injections as a technique to increase the duration of the block.[40,41] Sodium bicarbonate has also been used as an adjunct to shorten time to block onset in peripheral nerve blockade; however, precipitation when added to the local anesthetic can be problematic. Tramadol and midazolam are not recommended for peripheral nerve blockade because of their lack of efficacy and potential for neurotoxicity.

The Risks of Regional Anesthesia in Orthopedic Trauma

As shown in **Box 1** there are several risks specific to orthopedic trauma.

Compartment syndrome

Compartment syndrome is a condition in which swelling and increased pressure within a closed muscle compartment increases tissue pressure, compromising the

> **Box 1**
> **Risks of regional anesthesia in orthopedic trauma**
>
> Risks specific to the trauma
> - Preexisting hemodynamic instability
> - Specific preexisting medical condition
> - Existing coagulopathy
> - Uncooperative patient
> - Risk of masking compartment syndrome
> - Infection at the site of injection
>
> Technique-specific risks
>
> *Risks of neuraxial anesthesia*
> - Hemodynamic instability
> - Neurologic complications
> - Intravascular injection
> - Infection
>
> *Risks of peripheral nerve blocks*
> - Nerve injury
> - Infection
> - Intravascular injection

circulation and resulting in ischemia and muscle necrosis. More than 200,000 people are diagnosed annually with acute compartment syndrome in the United States,[42] with 40% of all cases resulting from tibial shaft fracture, 23% from soft tissue tibial trauma, and 18% from forearm fractures.[43] Possible causes of compartment syndrome are:

- Fractures
- Crush injuries
- Soft tissue trauma
- Intramedullary nailing
- Prolonged limb compression (eg, cast)
- Reperfusion injuries

The incidence of acute compartment syndrome is reported to be 4.3% in tibial shaft fractures, 3.1% with diaphyseal forearm fractures, and 0.25% in distal radius fractures.[44] The clinical presentation of compartment syndrome includes the following:

- Increased pain (unreliable sign)
- Paresthesia
- Pain on passive stretching of the affected limb
- Tense, hard muscle on palpation
- Loss of motor function (late sign)
- Ischemia (pulselessness; a late sign)

It is thought that postoperative pain control, especially regional anesthesia, may mask the symptoms of compartment syndrome and delay diagnosis. Because unrecognized and untreated compartment syndrome can result in permanent nerve damage within 8 hours, caution is needed when the possibility exist. It most commonly occurs in closed upper tibia fractures, with a small incidence occurring in forearm fractures. The injury is thought to be ischemic and, therefore, is humoral, as well as neural in nature. The nerve injury seems not to be caused by a total lack of blood supply because pulses are often present until the late stages. This ischemic pain is in addition to the initial incident and hence of a different nature, possibly because of the significant increase in hydrogen ion concentration as well as other factors in the area of ischemia. In case reports, one common theme was that a patient who has had a stable therapeutic analgesia and who suddenly experiences a significant increase in pain is very suspect. The close follow-up that includes, by necessity, attentive nursing care is imperative if a block is to be placed in these patients. There are no reported cases of missed compartment syndrome caused by effective regional analgesia in any recent military experiences provided that a high index of suspicion, ongoing patient assessment, and compartment pressure measurement were used.[45,46] Because of the low incidence, the issue of masking regional anesthesia is next to impossible to answer with a prospective, randomized, evidence-based study. Therefore regional analgesia has been relegated to case reports. However, Cometa and colleagues[47] described a case of compartment syndrome while the patient was receiving continuous peripheral femoral and sciatic nerve blocks. A more recent report by Munk-Andersen and Laustrup[48] presented another case of a successful diagnosis of compartment syndrome caused by breakthrough pain, despite a well-functioning CPNB. Kucera and Boezaart[49] reported 2 cases: one of ischemia discovered to be caused by a tight cast with a regional analgesia in place, and a case showing the different nature of ischemic pain in a 45-year-old woman with a history of diabetes mellitus, hypertension, and a 30-pack-year smoking history who presented with increasingly cold, cyanotic, and painful fingers in her right hand. She had necrotic lesions of her fourth and fifth fingers accompanied by severe ischemic type pain. A continuous C7 cervical paravertebral block was placed. Despite dense sensory and motor blockade, she still reported excruciating pain that ultimately required amputation because of her disease. Although this case was not secondary to trauma, it shows that, despite a neuroblockade, ischemic pain was identified.

Regional analgesia is often denied to patients with these injuries. Missed compartment syndrome occurs in patients without a block and patient controlled analgesia (PCA) analgesia. A report of 4 cases of tibia nailing with delayed diagnosis in patients with PCA shows that a PCA is not a safety net but diligent observation is the key to diagnosis.[50]

Recommendations on the use of regional anesthesia in patients at risk of compartment syndrome are given in **Table 2**.

Infection

Many practitioners are reluctant to perform a regional anesthetic technique in prehospital settings because of concern for infection. However, infectious complications with regional anesthesia are rare. When considering regional anesthesia in the prehospital setting it is important that the practitioner remember the following:

- Avoid performing blocks in patients with sepsis
- Avoid placing needles through an obvious skin infection
- Do not perform blocks in infected extremities
- Follow sterile precautions

The occurrence of infection related to the performance of single-shot nerve blocks has been reported to be between 0% and 3%, although most reports cite an incidence of less than 1%.[25] There are potentially greater risks associated with the CPNB

Table 2
Recommendations on the use of regional anesthesia in patients at risk of compartment syndrome

Type of Regional Anesthesia	Recommendation	Comments
Single-shot neuraxial	Yes	No reports; consider local anesthetics with shorter duration
Continuous spinal	No	Dense motor block
Continuous epidural	Yes	Monitor closely every 2 h to confirm sensation Consider low concentrations of local anesthetics; eg, 0.1% ropivacaine or 0.125%/0.0625% bupivacaine
Single-shot peripheral nerve block	Yes	Short-acting local anesthetic if risk is considered to be high
CPNB	Yes/no (risk/benefit decision)	Case reports only. Must have good observation of patient status throughout course of catheter. Make risk/benefit analysis

techniques than with single-shot techniques. One of the risks of continuous techniques is that catheters are frequently colonized (reported rate between 23% and 57%). However, clinical evidence of infection is uncommon (between 0% and 3% for CPNBs, <0.001% following spinal anesthesia, and <0.01% following epidural anesthesia).[51] Using meticulous technique and maximum barrier precautions, and tunneling the catheter best reduce the risk of infections. There is no evidence to support the routine use of preblock antibiotics for single-shot blocks or continuous nerve blocks, even though they do reduce colonization.[51] Colonization seems to be increased with frequent dressing changes.[52,53]

Risk factors for infectious complications with CPNBs include the following[53,54]:

- Duration of infusion greater than 48 hours
- Intensive care unit stay
- Axillary and femoral locations of the catheter
- Absence of antibiotic prophylaxis (possible)

Peripheral nerve injury
There is no evidence of increased incidence of nerve injury in patients with trauma compared with elective patients undergoing a block. Neurologic injury is one of the most serious complications of regional anesthesia. The incidence of transient adverse neurologic symptoms associated with CPNBs is 0 % to 1.4% for interscalene, 0.4% to 0.5% for femoral, and 0% to 1% for sciatic catheters.[54] Brull and colleagues[55] reviewed 32 studies published over a period of 10 years and concluded that the rate of neurologic complications after central nerve blocks is 0.04%, the rate of neuropathy after peripheral nerve blocks is 3%, and permanent neurologic injury is rare. In a retrospective study of 380,680 cases during a 10-year period, Welch and colleagues[56] found that perioperative nerve injury with regional anesthesia occurs more frequently when patients have a coexisting disease such as diabetes mellitus and hypertension or used tobacco. A neurologic deficit lasting longer than 6 weeks occurs in 0.2% of patients after regional anesthesia,[57] but most neurologic symptoms present at 4 to 6 weeks resolve spontaneously within 3 months of surgery.[54] Overall, neurologic deficits completely resolve within 2.6 years in most patients (71%) and an additional 26% experience partial recovery.[58] According to the American Society of

Anesthesiology Closed Claims Database,[59] lower extremity nerve injuries are rare and the most commonly injured peripheral nerves are as follows:

- Brachial plexus
- Median nerve
- Ulnar nerve
- Radial nerve

Permanent nerve injury is not completely preventable even in healthy patients receiving a competent standard of care. Before deciding on the use of a regional technique, a thorough documentation of the neurologic examination of the patient needs to be done. In addition, there should be a preprocedural discussion with all members of the team about risks and benefits in the particular situation. The American Society of Regional Anesthesia (ASRA) practice advisory on neurologic complications in regional anesthesia states the following[60]:

- There are no animal or human data to support the superiority of one nerve localization technique (paresthesia, nerve stimulation, ultrasonography) rather than another with regard to reducing the likelihood of nerve injury.
- There are no human data to support the superiority of one local anesthetic or additive rather than another, with regard to reducing the likelihood of neurotoxicity.
- Patients with diseased or previously injured nerves (eg, diabetes mellitus, severe peripheral vascular disease, chemotherapy) theoretically may be at an increased risk of neurologic injury. Although isolated case reports have been described, clinical experience can neither refute nor confirm these concerns. Careful risk/benefit assessment of regional anesthesia to alternative anesthesia and analgesia techniques should be considered.
- Patients with preexisting neurologic disease may be at the increased risk of new or worsening injury, regardless of the anesthetic technique. When regional anesthesia is thought to be appropriate for these patients, modifying the anesthetic technique may minimize potential risk.
- Based on a moderate amount of animal data, such modifications may include the use of less potent local anesthetic; minimizing local anesthetic dose, volume, and/or concentration; and avoiding or using a lower concentration of vasoactive additives. Limited human data neither confirm nor refute that these modifications are helpful.

Regional anesthesia in heavily sedated patients

One of the most controversial areas of regional anesthesia practice is whether or not to perform blocks on patients under heavy sedation or under general anesthesia. Proponents for performing blocks in only mildly sedated patients argue that such patients are able to communicate to the anesthesiologist the sensation of pain and thus lessen the likelihood of nerve injury. Proponents of performing blocks in anesthetized or heavily sedated patients argue that this practice brings the benefits of regional anesthesia to wider range of patients. At present, there is no hard evidence that regional anesthesia performed in patients under general anesthesia or deep sedation bears greater risk than when performed in lightly sedated patient. Thus, anesthesia providers are free to follow personal preferences. The ASRA recommendations for performing regional anesthesia in anesthetized or heavily sedated patients are[15]:

- The potential ability of general anesthesia or heavy sedation to obscure early signs of systemic local anesthetic toxicity is not a valid reason to forgo performing peripheral nerve blocks or epidural blocks in anesthetized or heavily sedated patients.

- There are no data to support the concept that peripheral nerve stimulation or ultrasonography and/or injection pressure monitoring reduce the risk of peripheral nerve injury in heavily sedated patients or patients under general anesthesia.
- General anesthesia or heavy sedation removes the ability of a patient to report warning signs, so regional anesthetic or pain blocks should not be performed with concurrent general anesthesia or heavy sedation in adults, except when the physician and patient conclude that the benefit clearly outweighs the risk.
- Because most reports of injury involve interscalene block in anesthetized patients, interscalene blocks should not be performed in anesthetized or heavily sedated patients.

Table 3	
Current guidelines of ASRA and Pain Medicine on neuraxial blockade in patients on antithrombotic or thrombolytic therapy	
Anticoagulant	**Guidelines**
UFH subcutaneous 500 units twice daily	No contraindication
UFH subcutaneous >10,000 units daily or >twice daily dosing	Not established
UFH IV (for vascular surgery)	Heparin 1 h after needle placement Remove catheter 2–4 h after last dose Reheparinize 1 h after catheter removal
LMWH (prophylactic low dose)	10–12 h after last dose First dose 6–8 h after operation 2 h after catheter removal for subsequent dose
LMWH (therapeutic dose)	24 h after last dose First dose 24 h after operation 2 h after catheter removal for subsequent dose
Warfarin	Stopped 4–5 d before INR normalized Catheter removal when INR <1.5
Aspirin	No contraindication
NSAIDs	No contraindication
Ticlopidine	14 d after last dose
Clopidogrel	7 d after last dose 5–7 d after last dose: document normalization of platelet function
Glycoprotein IIb/IIIa inhibitors	Avoid until platelet function recovered 24–48 h after abciximab 4–8 h after eptifibatide and tirofiban
Thrombin inhibitors (desirudin, lepirudin, bivalirudin, argatroban)	Contraindicated
Fondaparinux	Not established Perform under conditions used in clinical trials (single pass, atraumatic needle placement, avoid indwelling catheters)

Abbreviations: INR, International Normalized Ratio; IV, intravenously; LMWH, low-molecular-weight heparin; NSAIDs, nonsteroidal antiinflammatory drugs; UFH, unfractionated heparin.

Adapted from Horlocker TT, Wedel DJ, Rowlingson JC, et al. Regional anesthesia in the patient receiving antithrombotic or thrombolytic therapy: American Society of Regional Anesthesia and Pain Medicine evidence-based guidelines (third edition). Reg Anesth Pain Med 2010;35:64–101; with permission.

- Peripheral nerve blocks should not routinely be performed in most adults during general anesthesia or heavy sedation. However, the risk/benefit ratio should be considered, because it may improve the conditions of selected patients.
- Neurologic complications associated with regional anesthesia are rare, and particularly those complications that do not involve hematoma or infection.

Hemostasis in Trauma

Many patients with trauma are not placed on thromboprophylaxis in the initial period to avoid aggravation of potential bleeding in traumatized areas. Rib fractures are common in patients with trauma and may be treated with a thoracic epidural or paravertebral catheter. Paravertebral catheters are preferred by some clinicians because of the risk of epidural hematoma. Epidural hematoma is a rare but serious complication of epidural anesthesia. The current recommendations of the (third edition published in 2010) should be adhered to in anticoagulated patients. **Table 3** summarizes the current ASRA recommendations for neuraxial blockade in patients on antithrombotic or thrombolytic therapy. A thorough risk and benefit analysis must be made for each patient when considering neuraxial blockade.

For peripheral nerve blocks, the ASRA guidelines state, "For patients undergoing deep plexus or peripheral block, we recommend that guidelines regarding neuraxial techniques be similarly applied."[61] The Orthopedic Anesthesia, Pain, and Rehabilitation Society recently (2013) published a consensus that there is no evidence that the combination of thromboprophylaxis and peripheral nerve block increases the risk of major bleeding compared with either of the treatments alone. They furthermore concluded that, "Since both the performance of femoral nerve blocks and lumbar blocks combined with thromboprophylaxis were reported to be associated with retroperitoneal hematoma, the present review does not support the concept that deep and plexus blocks represent more of an increased risk of bleeding than superficial blocks in orthopedic patients receiving thromboprophylaxis."[62]

FUTURE CONSIDERATIONS AND SUMMARY

Patients with orthopedic trauma are often among the most complex cases for anesthesiologists because of associated comorbidities, the presence of multiple simultaneously existing injuries, the potential for multiple surgeries, and increased incidence of intraoperative complications. The benefits of regional anesthesia for the elective orthopedic patient are well established. The patients with orthopedic trauma have many additional considerations, in contrast with the elective surgical patient. The postoperative pain that patients with trauma experience can be in multiple locations; severe; and have the potential, when not treated adequately, to lead to other morbidities. There are additional complications with the overdependence on morphine as a primary pain therapy. Other results of inadequate pain relief include delayed rehabilitation of the orthopedic injury, delayed discharge, and predisposition for the development of chronic pain syndromes. Given their heightened inflammatory state and predisposition to infection, regional anesthetic techniques that decrease the pain and ultimate stress for orthopedic patients should be implemented wherever possible for this important subset of patients.

REFERENCES

1. National Trauma Institute. Trauma statistics. Available at: http://www.nationaltraumainstitute.org/home/trauma_statistics.html. Accessed February 12, 2014.

2. Wu JJ, Lollo L, Grabinsky A. Regional anesthesia in trauma medicine. Anesthesiol Res Pract 2011;2011:713281.
3. Bier A. Uber einen neuen weg lokalanesthesie an den gliedmassen zu erzeugen. Verhandlungen der Deutschen Gesellschaft fur Chirurgie 1908;27:204–14.
4. Ansbro FP. A method of continuous brachial plexus block. Am J Surg 1846;71: 716–22.
5. Corning J. Spinal anesthesia and local medication of the cord. New York Medical Journal 1885;42:493–5.
6. Bier A. Versuche über cocainisierung des rückenmarkes. Deutsche Zeitschrift für Chirurgie 1899;51:361–9.
7. Kent M, Upp J, Buckenmaier CC 3rd. Acute pain on and off the battlefield: what we do, what we know, and future directions. Int Anesthesiol Clin 2011;49:1–32.
8. Clark ME, Scholten JD, Walker RL, et al. Assessment and treatment of pain associated with combat-related polytrauma. Pain Med 2009;10:456–69.
9. Stojadinovic A, Auton A, Peoples GE, et al. Responding to challenges in modern combat casualty care: innovative use of advanced regional anesthesia. Pain Med 2006;7:330–8.
10. Buckenmaier C 3rd, Mahoney PF, Anton T, et al. Impact of an acute pain service on pain outcomes with combat-injured soldiers at Camp Bastion, Afghanistan. Pain Med 2012;13:919–26.
11. Buckenmaier CC 3rd, Rupprecht C, McKnight G, et al. Pain following battlefield injury and evacuation: a survey of 110 casualties from the wars in Iraq and Afghanistan. Pain Med 2009;10:1487–96.
12. Rosenberg A, Grande C, Bernstein R. Pain management and regional anesthesia in trauma. Philadelphia: WB Saunders; 2000.
13. Lenart MJ, Wong K, Gupta RK, et al. The impact of peripheral nerve techniques on hospital stay following major orthopedic surgery. Pain Med 2012;13:828–34.
14. Clark LD, Varbanova M. Regional anesthesia in trauma. In: Lake C, Johnson J, McLoughlin T, editors. Advances in anesthesia. Elsevier; 2009. p. 196–7.
15. Pavlov VA, Tracey KJ. The cholinergic anti-inflammatory pathway. Brain Behav Immun 2005;19:493–9.
16. Bierhaus A, Humpert PM, Nawroth PP. Linking stress to inflammation. Anesthesiol Clin 2006;24:325–40.
17. Memtsoudis SG, Sun X, Chiu YL, et al. Perioperative comparative effectiveness of anesthetic technique in orthopedic patients. Anesthesiology 2013;118:1046–58.
18. Benzon H, Rathmell J, Wu CL, et al. Practical management of pain. 5th edition. Philadelphia: Mosby; 2014.
19. Karmakar MK, Critchley LA, Ho AM, et al. Continuous thoracic paravertebral infusion of bupivacaine for pain management in patients with multiple fractured ribs. Chest 2003;123:424–31.
20. Morgan G, Mikhail M, Murray M. Clinical anesthesiology. 4th edition. McGraw-Hill; 2006. p. 284–5.
21. Urmey WF, Talts KH, Sharrock NE. One hundred percent incidence of hemidiaphragmatic paresis associated with interscalene brachial plexus anesthesia as diagnosed by ultrasonography. Anesth Analg 1991;72:498–503.
22. Chelly JE, Casati A, Al-Samsam T, et al. Continuous lumbar plexus block for acute postoperative pain management after open reduction and internal fixation of acetabular fractures. J Orthop Trauma 2003;17:362–7.
23. Newman B, McCarthy L, Thomas PW, et al. A comparison of pre-operative nerve stimulator-guided femoral nerve block and fascia iliaca compartment block in patients with a femoral neck fracture. Anaesthesia 2013;68:899–903.

24. Buckenmaier CC, McKnight GM, Winkley JV, et al. Continuous peripheral nerve block for battlefield anesthesia and evacuation. Reg Anesth Pain Med 2005;30: 202–5.

25. Ilfeld BM. Continuous peripheral nerve blocks: a review of the published evidence. Anesth Analg 2011;113:904–25.

26. Lai TT, Jaeger L, Jones BL, et al. Continuous peripheral nerve block catheter infections in combat-related injuries: a case report of five soldiers from Operation Enduring Freedom/Operation Iraqi Freedom. Pain Med 2011;12:1676–81.

27. Mariano ER, Cheng GS, Choy LP, et al. Electrical stimulation versus ultrasound guidance for popliteal-sciatic perineural catheter insertion: a randomized controlled trial. Reg Anesth Pain Med 2009;34:480–5.

28. Mariano ER, Loland VJ, Sandhu NS, et al. A trainee-based randomized comparison of stimulating interscalene perineural catheters with a new technique using ultrasound guidance alone. J Ultrasound Med 2010;29:329–36.

29. Bleckner L, Solla C, Fileta BB, et al. Serum free ropivacaine concentrations among patients receiving continuous peripheral nerve block catheters: is it safe for long-term infusions? Anesth Analg 2014;118:225–9.

30. Ilfeld BM, Moeller-Bertram T, Hanling SR, et al. Treating intractable phantom limb pain with ambulatory continuous peripheral nerve blocks: a pilot study. Pain Med 2013;14:935–42.

31. Bleckner LL, Bina S, Kwon KH, et al. Serum ropivacaine concentrations and systemic local anesthetic toxicity in trauma patients receiving long-term continuous peripheral nerve block catheters. Anesth Analg 2010;110:630–4.

32. Plunkett AR, Buckenmaier CC 3rd. Safety of multiple, simultaneous continuous peripheral nerve block catheters in a patient receiving therapeutic low-molecular-weight heparin. Pain Med 2008;9:624–7.

33. Manriquez RG, Pallares V. Continuous brachial plexus block for prolonged sympathectomy and control of pain. Anesth Analg 1978;57:128–30.

34. Berger A, Tizian C, Zenz M. Continuous plexus blockade for improved circulation in microvascular surgery. Ann Plast Surg 1985;14:16–9.

35. Loland VJ, Ilfeld BM, Abrams RA, et al. Ultrasound-guided perineural catheter and local anesthetic infusion in the perioperative management of pediatric limb salvage: a case report. Paediatr Anaesth 2009;19:905–7.

36. Ilfeld BM, Loland VJ, Gerancher JC, et al. The effects of varying local anesthetic concentration and volume on continuous popliteal sciatic nerve blocks: a dual-center, randomized, controlled study. Anesth Analg 2008;107:701–7.

37. Brummett CM, Williams BA. Additives to local anesthetics for peripheral nerve blockade. Int Anesthesiol Clin 2011;49:104–16.

38. Esmaoglu A, Yegenoglu F, Akin A, et al. Dexmedetomidine added to levobupivacaine prolongs axillary brachial plexus block. Anesth Analg 2010;111:1548–51.

39. Candido KD, Winnie AP, Ghaleb AH, et al. Buprenorphine added to the local anesthetic for axillary brachial plexus block prolongs postoperative analgesia. Reg Anesth Pain Med 2002;27:162–7.

40. Parrington SJ, O'Donnell D, Chan VW, et al. Dexamethasone added to mepivacaine prolongs the duration of analgesia after supraclavicular brachial plexus blockade. Reg Anesth Pain Med 2010;35:422–6.

41. Vieira PA, Pulai I, Tsao GC, et al. Dexamethasone with bupivacaine increases duration of analgesia in ultrasound-guided interscalene brachial plexus blockade. Eur J Anaesthesiol 2010;27:285–8.

42. Mannion S, Capdevila X. Acute compartment syndrome and the role of regional anesthesia. Int Anesthesiol Clin 2010;48:85–105.

43. Konstantakos EK, Dalstrom DJ, Nelles ME, et al. Diagnosis and management of extremity compartment syndromes: an orthopaedic perspective. Am Surg 2007; 73:1199–209.

44. Martin JT. Compartment syndromes: concepts and perspectives for the anesthesiologist. Anesth Analg 1992;75:275–83.

45. Clasper JC, Aldington DJ. Regional anaesthesia, ballistic limb trauma and acute compartment syndrome. J R Army Med Corps 2010;156:77–8.

46. Mar GJ, Barrington MJ, McGuirk BR. Acute compartment syndrome of the lower limb and the effect of postoperative analgesia on diagnosis. Br J Anaesth 2009; 102:3–11.

47. Cometa MA, Esch AT, Boezaart AP. Did continuous femoral and sciatic nerve block obscure the diagnosis or delay the treatment of acute lower leg compartment syndrome? A case report. Pain Med 2011;12:823–8.

48. Munk-Andersen H, Laustrup TK. Compartment syndrome diagnosed in due time by breakthrough pain despite continuous peripheral nerve block. Acta Anaesthesiol Scand 2013;57:1328–30.

49. Kucera TJ, Boezaart AP. Regional anesthesia does not consistently block ischemic pain: two further cases and a review of the literature. Pain Med 2014;15:316–9.

50. Richards H, Langston A, Kulkarni R, et al. Does patient controlled analgesia delay the diagnosis of compartment syndrome following intramedullary nailing of the tibia? Injury 2004;35:296–8.

51. Auroy Y, Benhamou D, Bargues L, et al. Major complications of regional anesthesia in France: the SOS regional anesthesia hotline service. Anesthesiology 2002;97:1274–80.

52. Morin AM, Kerwat KM, Klotz M, et al. Risk factors for bacterial catheter colonization in regional anaesthesia. BMC Anesthesiol 2005;5:1.

53. Capdevila X, Bringuier S, Borgeat A. Infectious risk of continuous peripheral nerve blocks. Anesthesiology 2009;110:182–8.

54. Capdevila X, Pirat P, Bringuier S, et al. Continuous peripheral nerve blocks in hospital wards after orthopedic surgery: a multicenter prospective analysis of the quality of postoperative analgesia and complications in 1,416 patients. Anesthesiology 2005;103:1035–45.

55. Brull R, McCartney CJ, Chan VW, et al. Neurological complications after regional anesthesia: contemporary estimates of risk. Anesth Analg 2007;104:965–74.

56. Welch MB, Brummett CM, Welch TD, et al. Perioperative peripheral nerve injuries: a retrospective study of 380,680 cases during a 10-year period at a single institution. Anesthesiology 2009;111:490–7.

57. Neuburger M, Breitbarth J, Reisig F, et al. Complications and adverse events in continuous peripheral regional anesthesia results of investigations on 3,491 catheters. Anaesthesist 2006;55:33–40 [in German].

58. Sviggum HP, Jacob AK, Mantilla CB, et al. Perioperative nerve injury after total shoulder arthroplasty: assessment of risk after regional anesthesia. Reg Anesth Pain Med 2012;37:490–4.

59. Liguori GA. Complications of regional anesthesia: nerve injury and peripheral neural blockade. J Neurosurg Anesthesiol 2004;16:84–6.

60. Neal JM, Bernards CM, Hadzic A, et al. ASRA practice advisory on neurologic complications in regional anesthesia and pain medicine. Reg Anesth Pain Med 2008;33:404–15.

61. Horlocker TT, Wedel DJ, Rowlingson JC, et al. Regional anesthesia in the patient receiving antithrombotic or thrombolytic therapy: American Society of Regional

Anesthesia and Pain Medicine evidence-based guidelines (third edition). Reg Anesth Pain Med 2010;35:64–101.

62. Chelly JE, Clark LD, Gebhard RE, et al. Consensus of the orthopedic anesthesia, pain, and rehabilitation society on the use of peripheral nerve blocks in patients receiving thromboprophylaxis. J Clin Anesth 2014;26:69–74.

Which Outcomes Related to Regional Anesthesia Are Most Important for Orthopedic Surgery Patients?

CrossMark

Ottokar Stundner, MD[a], Rainhold Ortmaier, MD[b],
Stavros G. Memtsoudis, MD, PhD[c],*

KEYWORDS

- Regional anesthesia • Outcomes • Pain management • Complications
- Economic advantages • Hospital stay • Functional outcome

KEY POINTS

- There is growing evidence that the use of regional anesthesia and analgesia contributes to improved outcomes in orthopedic patients with various important benefits for all stakeholders.
- Important short-term factors include comfort and adequate analgesia before, during and after the procedure; lack of unpleasant side effects; good operative conditions; optimized rehabilitation; a low complication profile; fast recovery; short hospital stay; and high patient satisfaction.
- Functional outcome is of extremely high importance to the patient as well as the practitioner because the primary goal of orthopedic surgery is the restoration or preservation of function and it ultimately constitutes an important determinant of the patients' quality of life.
- As evidenced by numerous available studies, regional anesthesia conveys many of these advantages and contributes to increased safety by decreasing complication incidence.
- Results with regard to the long-term functional impact of regional anesthesia are scarce and inconsistent at this time and high-quality research is warranted to more clearly define its role.

Conflict of Interest Statement: The authors certify that no relationships with commercial companies that have a direct financial interest in the subject matter or materials discussed in the article or with a company making a competing product exist.
[a] Department of Anesthesiology, Perioperative Medicine and Intensive Care Medicine, Paracelsus Medical University, Muellner Hauptstrasse 48, Salzburg 5020, Austria; [b] Department of Trauma Surgery and Sports Traumatology, Paracelsus Medical University, Muellner Hauptstrasse 48, Salzburg 5020, Austria; [c] Department of Anesthesiology, Hospital for Special Surgery, Weill Medical College of Cornell University, 535 East 70th Street, New York, NY 10021, USA
* Corresponding author.
E-mail address: memtsoudiss@hss.edu

INTRODUCTION

Regional anesthesia has gained considerable interest across virtually all surgical disciplines. Since the clinical introduction of local anesthetics in the 1800s, countless regional anesthetic techniques have been developed and popularized. The ability to provide analgesia in a selective fashion targeted specifically to surgical sites has led to the desire to increase knowledge about the mechanism of action as well as the subsequent effects associated with use of these techniques. Particularly for orthopedic surgery, regional anesthesia has come to constitute an indispensible part of the anesthesiologist's armamentarium. An increasing body of evidence documents the beneficial outcomes when regional anesthesia is applied.[1] Importantly, more focused and sustained pain control frequently obviates or reduces the need for systemic analgesic management. Beyond facilitated pain control, analgesic-related side effects such as respiratory and cardiovascular depression, gastrointestinal complications, sedation, and end-organ damage seem to be decreased.[2,3] These effects can prove critical in postoperative patients, allowing for the prevention of potentially life-threatening complications, improved patient comfort, and early mobilization. On a broader scale, regional anesthesia has been associated with a decrease in morbidity and mortality, particularly in patients with a high comorbidity burden and in the elderly.[4] Moreover, it has been linked to lower resource expenditure through earlier discharge, better short-term functional outcomes, lower rates of advanced service requirements (eg, critical care admission), transfusion need, and lower complication rates affecting virtually all organ systems. Importantly, all these effects have been observed while associated with very low risk for adverse events related to the regional anesthetics themselves.[5-7] However, there is considerable discussion as to which of these outcomes carry the most weight, either at the level of the individual patient or provider or from a healthcare management and public health perspective. This article briefly recapitulates recent literature pertaining to these subjects and presents an overview of various endpoints and their relevance, including pain management, morbidity and mortality, resource use, economic endpoints such as cost and length-of-stay, patient comfort and satisfaction, and functional outcomes.

PAIN MANAGEMENT

The most widely recognized indication of regional anesthesia and analgesia remains perioperative pain control.[8] Various techniques represent viable and frequently used approaches, particularly for analgesic management of orthopedic surgery on the extremities and pelvis, including major upper and lower extremity joint surgery, osteotomy and osteosynthesis, fracture treatment, and tumor and soft tissue surgery. It is less frequently used for spine surgical procedures but interest in regional anesthetic techniques in this population of patient is increasing.[9] It is obvious that various procedures are associated with sizable differences in invasiveness, spanning from diagnostic arthroscopies to simultaneous bilateral joint replacements or massive trauma, and are thus subject to different levels of pain, surgical stress, and impending complications. Due to their high use and drastically increasing demand,[10] total hip arthroplasty (THA) or total knee arthroplasty (TKA) are often chosen for comparative analyses of anesthetic techniques and associated outcomes including pain. In most studies, regional anesthesia is either compared with general anesthesia and systemic analgesia, or various regional anesthetic techniques are compared with each other. The spectrum of such approaches encompasses neuraxial analgesia (spinal, epidural, or combined spinal epidural anesthesia) as well as a large number of peripheral nerve blocks, either as a single injection or with insertion of a catheter at the injection site, allowing for prolonged administration of local anesthetic. The superior analgesic effect of central and peripheral regional anesthetic techniques for acute pain management has been demonstrated in countless studies and is reviewed extensively elsewhere.[8] Subjects undergoing total lower extremity joint replacement under general anesthesia were found to have disproportionately higher odds of experiencing moderate to severe postoperative pain (odds ratio [OR] = 8.51, CI 2.13–33.98) when compared with those receiving regional anesthesia in a review by Liu and colleagues.[11] Neuraxial techniques, as well as peripheral nerve blocks, have become an important constituent of almost any multimodal analgesic regimen in acute pain medicine across most surgical subspecialties. However, research into the optimal approaches to reach specific and nuanced goals is far from complete. The aim is to maximize analgesic efficacy and associated effects while minimizing potential for complications, neurologic impairment, or interference with recovery. Similarly, the impact of regional anesthesia on chronic pain development and its use in chronic pain treatment are not well-established. The outcome of chronic pain prevention may be of high importance in orthopedic patients. As a follow-up of the study mentioned above, Liu and colleagues[12] surveyed 1030 patients who underwent TKA or THA between 2006 and 2010 at 1 year after surgery using a standardized questionnaire for chronic postsurgical pain. Almost half (46%) reported persistent pain after these procedures (53% after TKA and 38% after THA). Risk factors for persistence of pain after 1 year included female sex, older age, previous hip or knee surgery, low-quality postoperative pain control, or presence of pain in other areas of the body. Importantly, subjects receiving general anesthesia had a 2.5 fold higher likelihood of a chronic pain outcome. Mechanisms proposed for reduction of hyperalgesia and development of persistent postsurgical pain invoked by regional anesthesia include a direct effect of local anesthetics,[13] anti-inflammatory effects,[14] prevention of opioid-induced hyperalgesia,[15] and central desensitization.[16] Moreover, regional anesthesia may facilitate the perioperative management of patients with a history of complex preexisting pain conditions.[17,18]

MORBIDITY, MORTALITY, AND COMPLICATIONS

The differential impact of regional anesthesia on the incidence of perioperative complications and mortality has been the subject of debate for decades. Although neuraxial techniques and peripheral nerve blocks have been used as the sole anesthetic or in conjunction with general anesthesia in orthopedic surgery for almost a century,[19] lack of hard evidence in a sufficiently powered cohort has left anesthesiologists and surgeons speculating about the magnitude of a suspected positive influence. Numerous, single-institution, relatively small trials have attempted to answer this question; however, most did not reach sufficient power to determine differences between the 2 approaches in terms of low-incidence outcomes such as major complications or mortality. Despite limitations, meta-analyses provided some insight into the subject. A systematic review of 28 such studies including 1538 subjects by Macfarlane and colleagues[20] confirmed that regional anesthesia is capable of reducing pain, morphine consumption, and opioid-related side effects, and it may decrease length-of-stay and facilitate rehabilitation. However, it failed to detect a difference in mortality, incidence of major cardiovascular complications, deep vein thrombosis, or pulmonary embolism. Other investigators analyzing larger sample sizes, on the other hand, show clear benefits in terms of major perioperative complications of neuraxial when compared with general anesthesia. In a general surgical population, a meta-analysis by Rodgers and colleagues,[21] including data from 141 studies (9599 subjects), evidenced a reduction in the incidence of mortality by 30% (OR=0.70, CI 0.54-0.90), and decreased rates of deep vein thrombosis; transfusion requirements; and respiratory, cardiac, and renal failure. However, the study did not detect variance between surgical subspecialties, likely due to lack of power. Similarly, Wijeysundera and colleagues[22] found benefits for neuraxial anesthesia in their large population-based study. They reported a slightly lower rate (1.7% vs 2.0%) and relative risk of 0.89 (CI 0.81-0.98, P = .02) of mortality when compared with general anesthesia. The effects seemed more pronounced in orthopedic and thoracic surgery than in other specialties. In a recent database study by Memtsoudis and colleagues,[23] 382,236 orthopedic subjects receiving neuraxial (11%) or general anesthesia (74.8%) or a combination of both techniques (14.2%) for total lower extremity joint replacement (THA or TKA) were analyzed. Use of regional anesthesia (neuraxial and combined neuraxial and general anesthesia) was associated with significantly lower incidences and adjusted OR for 30-day mortality when compared with general anesthesia alone (0.10%, 0.10% vs 0.18%, $P<.0001$; general vs neuraxial: OR = 1.83, CI 1.08–3.1, P = .0211; general vs combined general-neuraxial: OR = 1.70, CI 1.06–2.74, P = .0228). Moreover, the incidence and adjusted risk for numerous in-hospital complications, including cerebrovascular events, pulmonary compromise, cardiac complications, pneumonia, infectious complications, mechanical ventilation, and blood product transfusion, was significantly lower in groups receiving a form of regional anesthesia. Interestingly, those groups receiving a combination of regional and general anesthesia exhibited intermediate risk between the neuraxial-only (lowest risk) and general-only (highest risk) groups, suggesting that beneficial effects of neuraxial are not explainable by the avoidance of general anesthesia. Similar findings were obtained in subjects undergoing acute surgery for hip fracture. A study by Neuman and colleagues[24] found no difference in unadjusted rates of mortality after hip fracture surgery under general or regional anesthesia. However, after adjustment for age and comorbidities, clear benefits of regional anesthesia with regard to mortality and complications became apparent, suggesting a beneficial effect especially in patients who are elderly and less healthy. Although older patients, those with a particularly high comorbidity burden, or those subjected to high surgical acuity seem to benefit most from regional anesthesia, recent evidence suggests that decreased odds for major complications and resource use after total joint arthroplasty may be achievable across all age groups, irrespective of comorbidity prevalence.[25]

A caveat that must be kept in mind when discussing regional anesthesia outcomes is the risk for complications provoked by the technique itself, although risks for severely disabling long-term sequelae or infection were reported to be consistently low.[5] The incidence of nerve injury following total joint arthroplasty was reported to be 0.79% (CI 0.64%–0.96%) in TKA, and 0.72% (CI 0.58%–0.88%) in THA, with the risk for nerve injury remaining unchanged whether general, neuraxial anesthesia or peripheral nerve block were applied.[6,7] The incidence of spinal or epidural hematoma after central neuraxial blockade was similarly found to be low in a recent retrospective review by Pumberger and colleagues[26] examining more than 100,000 consecutive cases undergoing lower extremity joint replacement under central neuraxial anesthesia. The incidence of temporary epidural blood or gas collection confirmed by magnetic resonance tomography was 0.07 per 1.000 subjects (CI 0.02–0.13/1000), and persistent neurologic deficit did not occur.

RESOURCE USE: TRANSFUSION, CRITICAL CARE ADMISSION, VENTILATION

Highly invasive surgical procedures are frequently associated with significant blood loss. Despite a recent shift away from excessive allogeneic transfusion due to risk for complications[26] and high expense, the practice of blood transfusion can constitute a life-saving intervention after hemorrhage and still has a prominent place in orthopedic surgery. Alternative strategies have been explored, however, with varying success: blood product replenishment,[27] preoperative hematologic optimization,[27] antifibrinolytics,[28] and other measures to reduce perioperative blood loss. Regional anesthesia was identified as a contributor to reduced blood loss, effectively reducing the need for transfusions in many studies.[29,30] Moreover, patients undergoing major orthopedic surgery under regional anesthesia were found to require advanced services less frequently. An analysis by Memtsoudis and colleagues[31] determined risk factors for critical care service admission in approximately half a million total lower extremity joint arthroplasty recipients. Patients admitted to ICU incurred complications more frequently, had longer hospital stays and expenditure, and were less likely to be discharged home. Among the risk factors associated with need for critical care were advanced age, presence of cardiovascular complications, and, importantly, the anesthetic technique (neuraxial vs general: OR = 0.55, CI 0.51–0.60, $P<.0001$; combined neuraxial-general versus general: OR = 0.66, CI 0.61–0.71, $P<.0001$). A complication that frequently necessitates ICU admission is prolonged weaning from the respirator or requirement for postoperative mechanical ventilation. In the study in which the comparative impact of neuraxial versus general anesthesia on outcomes after THA or TKA was assessed, subjects receiving neuraxial or combined neuraxial-general anesthesia were less likely to require postoperative mechanical ventilation (THA: general vs neuraxial, OR = 1.57, CI 1.10–2.22, $P = .0085$; combined neuraxial-general vs general, OR = 1.49, CI 1.09–2.04, $P = .0091$; TKA: general vs neuraxial, OR = 1.72, 1.35,2.18, $P<.0001$; combined neuraxial-general vs general, OR = 1.32, CI 1.09–1.60, $P = .0021$).[23]

PATIENT COMFORT AND SATISFACTION

Intuitively, improved analgesia contributes to better patient comfort but, unless previous experiences with a similar surgery exist, direct comparison is often not possible for the individual patient. Patients' choice of an anesthetic technique is thus strongly influenced by either personal communications with former patients or from their own previous surgeries, with a positive experience being the strongest predictor for future preference for regional anesthesia.[32] Hence, the question of whether a patient would choose regional anesthesia again is considered a practical benchmark to grade satisfaction. Ironfield and colleagues[33] recently analyzed patient satisfaction data from an international registry of regional anesthesia. According to their data, 94.6% of patients (CI 94.0%–95.1%) who received a peripheral nerve block would undergo the procedure under regional anesthesia again. Whereas most (90%) patients felt adequately informed and cared for by their anesthesiologists, patients dissatisfied with either information provision or professional interaction were less willing to undergo a repeat nerve block. The investigators emphasize the importance of targeted physician-patient interaction through information and discussion of potential difficulties to improve patient comfort. Some discomfort can additionally arise during block placement, which is most frequently performed in the awake or only mildly sedated patient according to safety standards. Moreover, a significant fraction of patients were found to be afraid of hearing or seeing the surgery.[32] Appropriate education and/or sedation can alleviate both the discomfort associated with block placement as well as the surgical procedure itself and may be an important contributing factor to patient satisfaction.[34] In this context, it must be mentioned that advances in the use of ultrasound-guided approaches are replacing traditional, more painful or unpleasant means of nerve localization, including the (now scarcely practiced) paresthesia technique, leading to greater acceptance of regional anesthesia.[35]

ECONOMIC ADVANTAGES

From a healthcare economics standpoint, reductions in complication rates, lower incidence of advanced treatment necessity, and shorter hospital stay yield monetary benefits, although direct cost savings are challenging to quantify and even more challenging to compare between institutions or healthcare systems. Costs of regional anesthesia procedures are related to time, space, equipment, and training needed. However, it must be kept in mind that the direct cost difference of providing regional versus general anesthesia (eg, drugs, time spent for block establishment) is not well established, nor is it representative of the total economic benefit that can potentially be gained through outcome advantages. Again, although it is difficult to quantify these differences on a small scale, large comparative observational studies have shown benefits of regional anesthesia with regard to economic outcomes. In the study by Memtsoudis and colleagues[23] comparing outcomes of various types of anesthesia in THA and TKA recipients, median patient cost was higher in the neuraxial and combined neuraxial-general groups, when compared with the general group (15,366 [interquartile range (IQR) 12,733–18,240] US dollar [USD] vs 14,859 [IQR 12,607–17,676] vs 14,780 [IQR 12,120–18,500] USD, respectively; $P<.001$). However, the incidence of grossly increased individual patient cost (above the 75th percentile of all patients) was significantly lower in the groups receiving neuraxial anesthesia (21.4%) and combined neuraxial-general anesthesia (18.3%) compared with patients receiving general anesthesia only (23.4%, $P<.001$).

Duncan and colleagues[36] compared 100 subjects undergoing TKA or THA managed with a multimodal analgesic regimen (ie, a femoral nerve or posterior lumbar plexus catheter in addition to oral or intravenous opioid and nonopioid analgesics). These subjects were matched to a historic control group who did not receive the intervention. The estimated mean direct hospital costs were significantly lower in the group receiving regional anesthesia (difference 1999 USD; [CI 584–3231 USD], $P = .0004$), with the greatest impact among subjects with a high comorbidity burden. Interestingly, in another publication by Macario and McCoy[37] analyzing pharmacy cost of delivering analgesia to patients after joint replacement surgery under a multimodal analgesic regimen, the cost for analgesics amounts to only 1% of the total cost of surgery. Yet, almost two-thirds of these analgesics costs were for opioids, one-third for epidural local anesthetics, and only a small fraction for nonopioids. From these observations, a potential for savings by shifting analgesia away from the systemic route may be derived.

Among other factors, regional anesthesia has contributed to expedited release of patients from postoperative recovery areas.[38] Moreover, it has facilitated the performance of numerous orthopedic procedures in an outpatient setting,[39] with or without fast-track discharge, while preserving patient comfort.[40] Numerous reports show that even notoriously painful procedures such as open shoulder surgery are now frequently managed on an ambulatory basis. In a prospective study by Hadzic and colleagues,[41] 50 subjects were randomized to receive either fast-track general anesthesia with superficial bupivacaine wound infiltration or an interscalene brachial plexus block. Subjects in the regional anesthesia group were able to bypass the recovery area more frequently (76% vs 16%, $P<.001$), had lower pain scores, shorter recovery area stay (123 vs 286 minutes, $P<.001$), lower rates of hospital readmission (0 of 25 vs 4 of 25 cases, $P = .05$), and higher satisfaction with their care. Several practitioners leave perineural catheters in place and equip patients with a continuous infusion pump to take home,[42–46] with promising results.[47] For numerous other low-invasive outpatient orthopedic procedures, including knee arthroscopy,[48] anterior cruciate ligament reconstruction,[49] distal upper extremity surgery or carpal tunnel release,[50] regional anesthesia is superior to general anesthesia with regard to pain, earlier discharge, and better functional outcome in numerous publications. Anesthesia-controlled time is particularly reduced when dedicated induction areas or swing rooms are used for block establishment.[51] Mariano and colleagues[52] demonstrated significantly shorter anesthesia-controlled time in subject groups receiving upper extremity surgery with peripheral nerve blocks performed in an induction area, local anesthesia, or intravenous local anesthesia (Bier block) when compared with general anesthesia. Besides numerous other lower-invasive outpatient procedures such as joint arthroscopy or distal extremity surgery (eg, hallux valgus repair, hand joint procedures), attempts have been made to perform even knee arthroplasty in an ambulatory setting.[53] However, the effectiveness of such a step with regard to postdischarge complications and functional outcome remains to be determined.[54]

LENGTH-OF-STAY EARLIER DISCHARGE

Studies suggest that regional anesthesia is not only associated with decreased length of hospital stay for ambulatory surgery but also after inpatient procedures. A recent retrospective analysis by Lenart and colleagues[55] compared approximately 500 patients undergoing major orthopedic procedures receiving either traditional pain management (intravenous and/or oral narcotics), single injection peripheral nerve block, or continuous peripheral nerve blocks. Length-of-stay was shorter in both groups of patients receiving regional anesthesia. The investigators acknowledge that the magnitude of this effect was contingent on the surgical procedure performed and, therefore, stratified results using a Cox proportional hazard model, adjusting for type of surgery and other covariates (age, comorbidities, and American Society of Anesthesiologists [ASA] status). For the outcome of earlier hospital discharge, single peripheral nerve block versus no nerve block and continuous peripheral nerve block versus no nerve block yielded hazard ratios of 1.35 (CI 1.02–1.79) and 1.91 (CI 1.42–2.57), respectively. On average, patients receiving single-injection or continuous peripheral nerve blocks were 35% or 91% more likely to leave the hospital earlier than their counterparts receiving none of these interventions, independent of type of surgery and individual patient traits. A study examining the effects of a preemptive multimodal analgesic regimen using peripheral nerve blocks versus systemic analgesics conducted at the Mayo clinic (Mayo Clinic Total Joint Regional Anesthesia protocol) detected, besides lower complication rates and better pain control, earlier discharge capability (1.7 ± 1.9 days earlier, $P<.0001$) and shorter length-of-stay (3.8 vs 5.0 days, $P<.001$).[56] For neuraxial or combined neuraxial-general techniques, which are frequently applied in lower extremity total joint replacement surgery, the investigators similarly found shorter length-of-stay in approximately half a million patients undergoing THA or TKA compared with general anesthesia and lower incidence for length-of-stay exceeding the 75th percentile (neuraxial: 28.7%, neuraxial-general: 27.4%, general only: 35.4%, $P<.001$).[23]

IMPROVED FUNCTIONAL OUTCOME AND INPATIENT FALL RISK

Functional outcome is of extremely high importance to the patient as well as the orthopedic surgeon because the primary goal of orthopedic surgery is the restoration or preservation of function. The ability to perform tasks in everyday life or beyond (eg, participation in sports) is an important determinant of patients' quality of life. Type of surgery and the extent of preexisting disability are most strongly related to postoperative outcome.[57] However, the impact of different anesthetic and analgesic regimens on functional outcome is still subject to intense controversy because available evidence is scarce and conflicting. Various performance-based scores, measurements, and self-reported functioning in the short-term, as well as the long-term, define functional results after orthopedic surgery. Measures used to objectively quantify performance-based outcomes comprise range of motion (ROM) tests, maximum voluntary isometric contraction, ambulation, and handwork scores. These include walking for a defined time, stair climbing, and time-up-and-go measures (the time required to rise from a chair, walk 3 m, return to the chair and sit down again). Subjective measures include self-reported outcomes such as the Short Musculoskeletal Function Assessment (SMFA), the Western Ontario McMaster (WOMAC) Osteoarthritis Index, Constant Murley Score, the Knee Society evaluation, the Community Health Activities Model Program for Seniors (CHAMPS), or, for the upper extremity, the Disability of the Arm, Shoulder and Hand (DASH) questionnaire.[58] Jeske and colleagues[59] compared regional anesthesia (suprascapular nerve block) with placebo and local subacromial infiltration in 45 subjects undergoing arthroscopic subacromial decompression. The nerve block group achieved significantly better ROM levels along with higher satisfaction and lower pain scores, when compared with the placebo or local infiltration groups. Other studies similarly report improved ROM, faster attainment of physical therapy goals, earlier ambulation, and more effective rehabilitation due to less pain when central or peripheral regional anesthesia was used; however, the long-term benefits were far less convincing.[58,60,61] In subjects receiving lower extremity orthopedic surgery, effects seemed even less pronounced when some of the measurements mentioned previously were applied.[62–69] Although available evidence consistently shows lower pain scores in patients managed with regional versus systemic analgesia, minimal to no differences can be detected with regard to functional outcomes. However, many of the available functional outcome-centric studies should be interpreted with caution because they are limited by small sample sizes, compare a wide variety of regional anesthetic as well as surgical techniques to each other, are biased by subjective measurements, or only poorly account for preexisting disability.

One specific concern frequently voiced among perioperative clinicians, especially those with knee arthroplasty patients, is inpatient falls. Some investigators have suggested that the use of peripheral nerve blocks may be associated with increased fall risk due to the associated motor weakness produced by such techniques.[70] However, a recent large population-based study analyzing the independent impact of peripheral nerve blockade on the risk of falling while in the hospital did not find any association in this real-world setting. This is likely because successful use of peripheral nerve blocks is often associated with various fall prevention programs to effectively address this complication. Interestingly, the use of neuraxial versus general anesthesia decreased the risk for inpatient falls by approximately 25%, possibly by decreasing the need for systemic opioids and other anesthetic agents with the propensity to alter sensorium.[71] Other investigators have suggested that catheter techniques may be more likely to lead to fall risk than single-injection approaches,[70] thus pointing out the importance of more research into related mechanisms. Further, an increasing number of investigators are seeking to find regional anesthetic approaches that minimize motor dysfunction while providing adequate pain relief. In this context, investigators have suggested that the use of saphenous, as compared with femoral, nerve blocks may indeed achieve this goal.[72,73]

SUMMARY

Regional anesthesia and analgesia may provide benefits in terms of a wide range of medical and economic outcomes, as evidenced by numerous available studies. Regional anesthetic techniques convey many intrinsic advantages and actively contribute to increased safety by decreasing complication incidence and mortality. This holds particularly true in patients with a higher comorbidity burden or the elderly but is not limited to these groups. In the long term, functional outcome plays a major role for all parties involved. A function after orthopedic surgery is an important parameter of patients' quality of life. Lack thereof frequently necessitates long-term analgesic requirements, subsequent procedures or revisions, exposing patient to disability, drug side effects, and other associated risks. Unfortunately, results for the long-term functional impact of regional anesthesia are scarce and inconsistent at this time. Studies using standardized anesthetic and surgical approaches, placing focus on clinically meaningful and objective outcome measures, adequate assessment intervals, and adjustment for individual and practitioner differences may provide insight into this complex subject.[74] Such research is clearly warranted to explore long-term benefits of regional anesthesia. However, advantages in short-term and intermediate-term pain management, reduction of complication incidence, and economic benefits make regional anesthesia an effective and elegant modality for orthopedic procedures.

REFERENCES

1. Chelly JE, Ben-David B, Williams BA, et al. Anesthesia and postoperative analgesia: outcomes following orthopedic surgery. Orthopedics 2003;26: s865–71.
2. Richman JM, Liu SS, Courpas G, et al. Does continuous peripheral nerve block provide superior pain control to opioids? A meta-analysis. Anesth Analg 2006; 102:248–57.
3. Stundner O, Memtsoudis SG. Regional anesthesia and analgesia in critically ill patients: a systematic review. Reg Anesth Pain Med 2012;37:537–44.
4. Stundner O, Danninger T, Memtsoudis SG. Regional anesthesia in patients with significant comorbid disease. Minerva Anestesiol 2013;79:1281–90.
5. Capdevila X, Pirat P, Bringuier S, et al. Continuous peripheral nerve blocks in hospital wards after orthopedic surgery: a multicenter prospective analysis of the quality of postoperative analgesia and complications in 1,416 patients. Anesthesiology 2005;103:1035–45.
6. Jacob AK, Mantilla CB, Sviggum HP, et al. Perioperative nerve injury after total hip arthroplasty: regional anesthesia risk during a 20-year cohort study. Anesthesiology 2011;115:1172–8.
7. Jacob AK, Mantilla CB, Sviggum HP, et al. Perioperative nerve injury after total knee arthroplasty: regional anesthesia risk during a 20-year cohort study. Anesthesiology 2011;114:311–7.
8. Boezaart AP, Munro AP, Tighe PJ. Acute pain medicine in anesthesiology. F1000Prime Rep 2013;5:54.
9. De Rojas JO, Syre P, Welch WC. Regional anesthesia versus general anesthesia for surgery on the lumbar spine: a review of the modern literature. Clin Neurol Neurosurg 2014;119C:39–43.
10. Kurtz S, Ong K, Lau E, et al. Projections of primary and revision hip and knee arthroplasty in the United States from 2005 to 2030. J Bone Joint Surg Am 2007;89:780–5.

11. Liu SS, Buvanendran A, Rathmell JP, et al. Predictors for moderate to severe acute postoperative pain after total hip and knee replacement. Int Orthop 2012;36:2261–7.

12. Liu SS, Buvanendran A, Rathmell JP, et al. A cross-sectional survey on prevalence and risk factors for persistent postsurgical pain 1 year after total hip and knee replacement. Reg Anesth Pain Med 2012;37:415–22.

13. Barreveld A, Witte J, Chahal H, et al. Preventive analgesia by local anesthetics: the reduction of postoperative pain by peripheral nerve blocks and intravenous drugs. Anesth Analg 2013;116:1141–61.

14. Beloeil H, Ji RR, Berde CB. Effects of bupivacaine and tetrodotoxin on carrageenan-induced hind paw inflammation in rats (Part 2): cytokines and p38 mitogen-activated protein kinases in dorsal root ganglia and spinal cord. Anesthesiology 2006;105:139–45.

15. Meleine M, Rivat C, Laboureyras E, et al. Sciatic nerve block fails in preventing the development of late stress-induced hyperalgesia when high-dose fentanyl is administered perioperatively in rats. Reg Anesth Pain Med 2012;37:448–54.

16. Rivat C, Bollag L, Richebe P. Mechanisms of regional anaesthesia protection against hyperalgesia and pain chronicization. Curr Opin Anaesthesiol 2013. [Epub ahead of print].

17. Souzdalnitski D, Halaszynski TM, Faclier G. Regional anesthesia and co-existing chronic pain. Curr Opin Anaesthesiol 2010;23:662–70.

18. Tumber PS. Optimizing perioperative analgesia for the complex pain patient: medical and interventional strategies. Can J Anaesth 2014;61:131–40.

19. Mulroy MA. History of regional anesthesia. In: Eger E, Saidman L, Westhorpe R, editors. The wondrous story of anesthesia. New York: Springer; 2014. p. 859–70.

20. Macfarlane AJ, Prasad GA, Chan VW, et al. Does regional anesthesia improve outcome after total knee arthroplasty? Clin Orthop Relat Res 2009;467:2379–402.

21. Rodgers A, Walker N, Schug S, et al. Reduction of postoperative mortality and morbidity with epidural or spinal anaesthesia: results from overview of randomised trials. BMJ 2000;321:1493.

22. Wijeysundera DN, Beattie WS, Austin PC, et al. Epidural anaesthesia and survival after intermediate-to-high risk noncardiac surgery: a population-based cohort study. Lancet 2008;372:562–9.

23. Memtsoudis SG, Sun X, Chiu YL, et al. Perioperative comparative effectiveness of anesthetic technique in orthopedic patients. Anesthesiology 2013;118:1046–58.

24. Neuman MD, Silber JH, Elkassabany NM, et al. Comparative effectiveness of regional versus general anesthesia for hip fracture surgery in adults. Anesthesiology 2012;117:72–92.

25. Memtsoudis SG, Rasul R, Suzuki S, et al. Does the impact of the type of anesthesia on outcomes differ by patient age and comorbidity burden? Reg Anesth Pain Med 2014;39:112–9.

26. Pumberger M, Memtsoudis SG, Stundner O, et al. An analysis of the safety of epidural and spinal neuraxial anesthesia in more than 100,000 consecutive major lower extremity joint replacements. Reg Anesth Pain Med 2013;38:515–9.

27. So-Osman C, Nelissen RG, Koopman-van Gemert AW, et al. Patient blood management in elective total hip- and knee-replacement surgery (part 2): a randomized controlled trial on blood salvage as transfusion alternative using a restrictive transfusion policy in patients with a preoperative hemoglobin above 13 g/dl. Anesthesiology 2014;120:852–60.

28. Ido K, Neo M, Asada Y, et al. Reduction of blood loss using tranexamic acid in total knee and hip arthroplasties. Arch Orthop Trauma Surg 2000;120:518–20.

29. Guay J. The effect of neuraxial blocks on surgical blood loss and blood transfusion requirements: a meta-analysis. J Clin Anesth 2006;18:124–8.
30. Park JH, Rasouli MR, Mortazavi SM, et al. Predictors of perioperative blood loss in total joint arthroplasty. J Bone Joint Surg Am 2013;95:1777–83.
31. Memtsoudis SG, Sun X, Chiu YL, et al. Utilization of critical care services among patients undergoing total hip and knee arthroplasty: epidemiology and risk factors. Anesthesiology 2012;117:107–16.
32. Dove P, Gilmour F, Weightman WM, et al. Patient perceptions of regional anesthesia: influence of gender, recent anesthesia experience, and perioperative concerns. Reg Anesth Pain Med 2011;36:332–5.
33. Ironfield CM, Barrington MJ, Kluger R, et al. Are patients satisfied after peripheral nerve blockade? Results from an International Registry of Regional Anesthesia. Reg Anesth Pain Med 2014;39:48–55.
34. Hohener D, Blumenthal S, Borgeat A. Sedation and regional anaesthesia in the adult patient. Br J Anaesth 2008;100:8–16.
35. Luyet C, Constantinescu M, Waltenspul M, et al. Transition from nerve stimulator to sonographically guided axillary brachial plexus anesthesia in hand surgery: block quality and patient satisfaction during the transition period. J Ultrasound Med 2013;32:779–86.
36. Duncan CM, Hall Long K, Warner DO, et al. The economic implications of a multimodal analgesic regimen for patients undergoing major orthopedic surgery: a comparative study of direct costs. Reg Anesth Pain Med 2009;34:301–7.
37. Macario A, McCoy M. The pharmacy cost of delivering postoperative analgesia to patients undergoing joint replacement surgery. J Pain 2003;4:22–8.
38. Williams BA, Kentor ML. The WAKE(c) score: patient-centered ambulatory anesthesia and fast-tracking outcomes criteria. Int Anesthesiol Clin 2011;49:33–43.
39. Chelly JE, Gebhard R, Greger J, et al. Regional anesthesia for outpatient orthopedic surgery. Minerva Anestesiol 2001;67:227–32.
40. Moore JG, Ross SM, Williams BA. Regional anesthesia and ambulatory surgery. Curr Opin Anaesthesiol 2013;26:652–60.
41. Hadzic A, Williams BA, Karaca PE, et al. For outpatient rotator cuff surgery, nerve block anesthesia provides superior same-day recovery over general anesthesia. Anesthesiology 2005;102:1001–7.
42. Boezaart AP. Continuous interscalene block for ambulatory shoulder surgery. Best Pract Res Clin Anaesthesiol 2002;16:295–310.
43. Faryniarz D, Morelli C, Coleman S, et al. Interscalene block anesthesia at an ambulatory surgery center performing predominantly regional anesthesia: a prospective study of one hundred thirty-three patients undergoing shoulder surgery. J Shoulder Elbow Surg 2006;15:686–90.
44. Fredrickson MJ, Ball CM, Dalgleish AJ. Successful continuous interscalene analgesia for ambulatory shoulder surgery in a private practice setting. Reg Anesth Pain Med 2008;33:122–8.
45. Lin E, Choi J, Hadzic A. Peripheral nerve blocks for outpatient surgery: evidence-based indications. Curr Opin Anaesthesiol 2013;26:467–74.
46. Nielsen KC, Greengrass RA, Pietrobon R, et al. Continuous interscalene brachial plexus blockade provides good analgesia at home after major shoulder surgery-report of four cases. Can J Anaesth 2003;50:57–61.
47. Salviz EA, Xu D, Frulla A, et al. Continuous interscalene block in patients having outpatient rotator cuff repair surgery: a prospective randomized trial. Anesth Analg 2013;117:1485–92.

48. Casati A, Cappelleri G, Berti M, et al. Randomized comparison of remifentanil-propofol with a sciatic-femoral nerve block for out-patient knee arthroscopy. Eur J Anaesthesiol 2002;19:109–14.

49. Williams BA, Kentor ML, Williams JP, et al. Process analysis in outpatient knee surgery: effects of regional and general anesthesia on anesthesia-controlled time. Anesthesiology 2000;93:529–38.

50. Gebhard RE, Al-Samsam T, Greger J, et al. Distal nerve blocks at the wrist for outpatient carpal tunnel surgery offer intraoperative cardiovascular stability and reduce discharge time. Anesth Analg 2002;95:351–5 table of contents.

51. Head SJ, Seib R, Osborn JA, et al. A "swing room" model based on regional anesthesia reduces turnover time and increases case throughput. Can J Anaesth 2011;58:725–32.

52. Mariano ER, Chu LF, Peinado CR, et al. Anesthesia-controlled time and turnover time for ambulatory upper extremity surgery performed with regional versus general anesthesia. J Clin Anesth 2009;21:253–7.

53. Berger RA, Kusuma SK, Sanders SA, et al. The feasibility and perioperative complications of outpatient knee arthroplasty. Clin Orthop Relat Res 2009;467:1443–9.

54. Cross MB, Berger R. Feasibility and safety of performing outpatient unicompartmental knee arthroplasty. Int Orthop 2014;38:443–7.

55. Lenart MJ, Wong K, Gupta RK, et al. The impact of peripheral nerve techniques on hospital stay following major orthopedic surgery. Pain Med 2012;13:828–34.

56. Hebl JR, Dilger JA, Byer DE, et al. A preemptive multimodal pathway featuring peripheral nerve block improves perioperative outcomes after major orthopedic surgery. Reg Anesth Pain Med 2008;33:510–7.

57. Hawker GA, Badley EM, Borkhoff CM, et al. Which patients are most likely to benefit from total joint arthroplasty? Arthritis Rheum 2013;65:1243–52.

58. Bernucci F, Carli F. Functional outcome after major orthopedic surgery: the role of regional anesthesia redefined. Curr Opin Anaesthesiol 2012;25:621–8.

59. Jeske HC, Kralinger F, Wambacher M, et al. A randomized study of the effectiveness of suprascapular nerve block in patient satisfaction and outcome after arthroscopic subacromial decompression. Arthroscopy 2011;27:1323–8.

60. Egol KA, Soojian MG, Walsh M, et al. Regional anesthesia improves outcome after distal radius fracture fixation over general anesthesia. J Orthop Trauma 2012;26:545–9.

61. McCartney CJ, Brull R, Chan VW, et al. Early but no long-term benefit of regional compared with general anesthesia for ambulatory hand surgery. Anesthesiology 2004;101:461–7.

62. Carli F, Clemente A, Asenjo JF, et al. Analgesia and functional outcome after total knee arthroplasty: periarticular infiltration vs continuous femoral nerve block. Br J Anaesth 2010;105:185–95.

63. Charous MT, Madison SJ, Suresh PJ, et al. Continuous femoral nerve blocks: varying local anesthetic delivery method (bolus versus basal) to minimize quadriceps motor block while maintaining sensory block. Anesthesiology 2011;115: 774–81.

64. Fetherston CM, Ward S. Relationships between post operative pain management and short term functional mobility in total knee arthroplasty patients with a femoral nerve catheter: a preliminary study. J Orthop Surg Res 2011;6:7.

65. Holm B, Kristensen MT, Myhrmann L, et al. The role of pain for early rehabilitation in fast track total knee arthroplasty. Disabil Rehabil 2010;32:300–6.

66. Ilfeld BM, Shuster JJ, Theriaque DW, et al. Long-term pain, stiffness, and functional disability after total knee arthroplasty with and without an extended

ambulatory continuous femoral nerve block: a prospective, 1-year follow-up of a multicenter, randomized, triple-masked, placebo-controlled trial. Reg Anesth Pain Med 2011;36:116–20.

67. Jordan C, Davidovitch RI, Walsh M, et al. Spinal anesthesia mediates improved early function and pain relief following surgical repair of ankle fractures. J Bone Joint Surg Am 2010;92:368–74.

68. Ong JC, Chin PL, Fook-Chong SM, et al. Continuous infiltration of local anaesthetic following total knee arthroplasty. J Orthop Surg (Hong Kong) 2010;18:203–7.

69. Paul JE, Arya A, Hurlburt L, et al. Femoral nerve block improves analgesia outcomes after total knee arthroplasty: a meta-analysis of randomized controlled trials. Anesthesiology 2010;113:1144–62.

70. Ilfeld BM, Duke KB, Donohue MC. The association between lower extremity continuous peripheral nerve blocks and patient falls after knee and hip arthroplasty. Anesth Analg 2010;111:1552–4.

71. Memtsoudis SG, Danninger T, Rasul R, et al. Inpatient falls after total knee arthroplasty: the role of anesthesia type and peripheral nerve blocks. Anesthesiology 2014;120:551–63.

72. Jaeger P, Nielsen ZJ, Henningsen MH, et al. Adductor canal block versus femoral nerve block and quadriceps strength: a randomized, double-blind, placebo-controlled, crossover study in healthy volunteers. Anesthesiology 2013;118:409–15.

73. Kim DH, Lin Y, Goytizolo EA, et al. Adductor canal block versus femoral nerve block for total knee arthroplasty: a prospective, randomized, controlled trial. Anesthesiology 2014;120:540–50.

74. Choi S, Trang A, McCartney CJ. Reporting functional outcome after knee arthroplasty and regional anesthesia: a methodological primer. Reg Anesth Pain Med 2013;38:340–9.

Optimizing Perioperative Care for Patients with Hip Fracture

Jiabin Liu, MD, PhD[a],*, Jaimo Ahn, MD, PhD[b],
Nabil M. Elkassabany, MD, MSCE[a]

KEYWORDS

- Hip fracture • Perioperative care • Optimization • Algorithm

KEY POINTS

- Hip fracture surgery is semi-urgent in nature, and is associated with significant morbidity and mortality in comparison with elective hip surgery.
- Hip fracture surgery should be performed within 24 to 48 hours after admission.
- Institutional guidelines are recommended to improve efficiency.
- The focus of preoperative preparation is risk assessment, stratification, and management to achieve effective and efficient optimization within 48 hours or sooner.
- The optimization process should extend throughout the whole perioperative period.

THE CHALLENGES

Hip fracture is one of the most common orthopedic conditions associated with significant morbidity and mortality. It is estimated that there were 1.66 million hip fractures worldwide in 1990, projected to be more than 6 million by the year 2050.[1]

Hip fracture surgery is usually defined as intermediate-risk procedure. However, patients with hip fracture are usually older with significant comorbidities, which place them in a much higher risk category with regard to perioperative morbidity and mortality.[2–4]

Although hip fracture surgery is a semi-urgent procedure by nature, delayed surgical treatment could cause a downward spiral with a poor outcome. Meta-analysis on 257,367 patients indicated that operative delay beyond 48 hours after admission is associated with 41% higher 30-day all-cause mortality and 32% higher 1-year all-cause mortality.[5] It is thus generally recommended that patients with a hip fracture

[a] Department of Anesthesiology and Critical Care, Perelman School of Medicine, University of Pennsylvania, Philadelphia, PA 19104, USA; [b] Department of Orthopedic Surgery, Perelman School of Medicine, University of Pennsylvania, Philadelphia, PA 19104, USA
* Corresponding author. Department of Anesthesiology and Critical Care, University of Pennsylvania, 319C John Morgan Building, 3400 Spruce Street, Philadelphia, PA 19104.
E-mail address: Jiabin.Liu@uphs.upenn.edu

Anesthesiology Clin 32 (2014) 823–839
http://dx.doi.org/10.1016/j.anclin.2014.08.010
1932-2275/14/$ – see front matter © 2014 Elsevier Inc. All rights reserved.

anesthesiology.theclinics.com

should undergo surgery as soon as possible once the patient's medical condition is optimized.[6] Hereby clinicians are presented with the challenge to optimize the complex patient within a short time period.

PREOPERATIVE RISK CONSIDERATION AND OPTIMIZATION
Cardiac Consideration in Patients with Hip Fracture and Risk Stratification

Cardiac risk for elective hip surgery is generally treated as intermediate risk, with a 30-day cardiac complication rate of 1% to 5%.[7] This estimation is based on an elective, relatively young and healthy patient population. However, patients with hip fracture are usually older, with significant cardiac and pulmonary comorbidities. Repair surgery for a hip fracture is also considered semi-urgent. Lawrence and colleagues[3] analyzed close to 9000 patients 60 years or older undergoing hip fracture surgery, and reported that 8% of patients had cardiac complications postoperatively. The 30-day and 1-year mortality was 4% and 16%, respectively.

Nonetheless, the benefit of hip fracture surgery usually outweighs the perioperative risks. The goal is to optimize the patient's cardiac condition within a short period of time. The American College of Cardiology (ACC) and the American Heart Association (AHA) have published a stepwise approach for cardiac assessment preoperatively in noncardiac patients.[7,8] The stepwise approach is helpful in determining the readiness for surgery and identifying the necessity of further medical management. The ACC/AHA guidelines consist of 7 steps with consideration of the emergency nature of the surgery, active cardiac condition, surgical risk, functional capacity of the patient, and clinical risk factor stratification when the previous steps are unable to lead to a favorable decision.[7,8]

There are several characteristic features of hip fractures. First, they are usually considered semi-urgent procedures, except the open hip fracture, which would be considered emergent. Second, patients with hip fracture are usually older, with substantial comorbidities and limited baseline functional capacity. A complete history and physical examination should be performed on all patients, while understanding that this is challenging for patients with mental status changes either at baseline or due to the acute event. Sometimes additional tests may be indicated, thus delaying the timing of surgery.

In consideration of these specific features, the authors propose a modified algorithm to guide the management of patients with hip fracture (**Fig. 1**).

Step 1. The physician should determine the emergent/urgent nature of the surgery. Complete history and physical examination should be performed. All necessary treatment should be initiated to maximally resuscitate and stabilize patients with regard to acute blood loss, fluid deficiency, coexisting injuries, and so forth.

Step 2. Does the patient have active cardiac conditions? There are 4 groups of active cardiac conditions that warrant further investigation: unstable coronary syndromes, decompensated heart failure defined as New York Heart Association functional class IV, worsening or new-onset heart failure, significant arrhythmia, and severe valvular disease.[7,9] Patients with 1 or more of these active cardiac conditions may require further evaluation and treatment. Hospitalists and cardiologists can be helpful in optimizing patients in a timely manner and should be consulted as needed. The goal of consultation is to determine the severity of the medical condition and identify any potentially modifiable factors for improvement. Even though some of the desired treatments might not achieve maximum benefit preoperatively, their continuation throughout the perioperative period should target the best positive outcome for those patients with hip fracture.

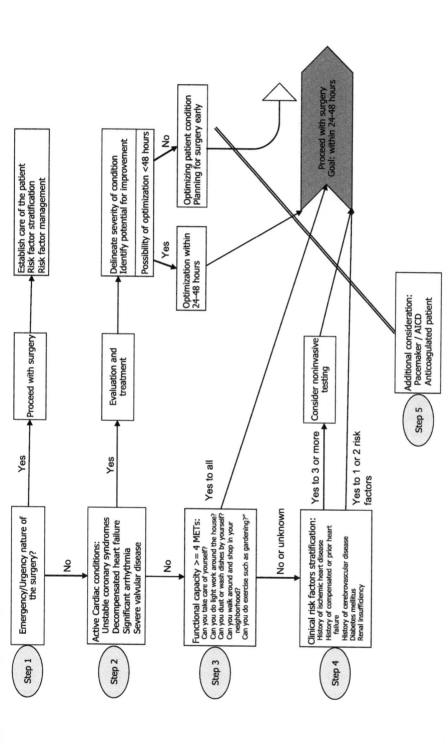

Fig. 1. Cardiac evaluation and care algorithm for patients with hip fracture. The algorithm is modified for patients with hip fracture based on American College of Cardiology/American Heart Association 2007/2014 guideline on perioperative cardiovascular evaluation and care for noncardiac surgery. AICD, automatic implantable cardioverter-defibrillator; MET, metabolic equivalents.

Patients with hip fracture and recent myocardial infarction (<1 month previously) had a significantly high incidence of mortality of 45.4% and 63.5% at 1 and 6 months, respectively.[10] The decision to proceed with surgical treatment should be made cautiously with such a high incidence of mortality. A collaborative decision should be made between patient, caregiver, anesthesiologist, surgeon, and other team members. Patients with heart failure were also associated with worse surgical outcomes.[11,12] Significant valvular disease, especially aortic stenosis, is relatively common in the geriatric population,[13,14] and contributes to severe cardiac complications.[9,15–19] It is recommended that an echocardiogram be performed for patients with suspected valvular disease preoperatively to guide perioperative management.[20] Cardiac intervention is rarely advised before the repair surgery for hip fracture. However, there are limited data to provide guidance for treatment priority.

Step 3. Does the patient have a functional capacity at 4 metabolic equivalents (METs) or higher without any symptoms? The patient will meet the minimal criteria on functional capacity if answering "yes" to all these questions (adopted from Fleisher and colleagues[8]), including:

"Can you take care of yourself?"
"Can you do light work around the house?"
"Can you dust or wash dishes by yourself?"
"Can you walk around and shop in your neighborhood?"
"Can you do exercise such as gardening?"

Although the METs evaluation is fairly simple, it reliably predicts the risks of perioperative and long-term cardiac complications.[21–24] Surgery should proceed if the patient with hip fracture has 4 or more METs and is without any active cardiac condition.

Step 4. If the patient has less than 4 METs or is unable to be evaluated for functional capacity, clinical risk factors should be considered before making a decision as to whether surgery should proceed or an additional workup is indicated. These 5 clinical risk factors are history of ischemic heart disease, history of compensated or prior heart failure, history of cerebrovascular disease, diabetes mellitus, and renal insufficiency. Although the ACC and AHA both recommend proceeding with surgery even in the presence of these risk factors because of the intermediate-risk nature of hip fracture repair, it is important to emphasize heart rate control and close hemodynamic management during the perioperative period, especially for patients with 3 or more risk factors.[21–24]

Step 5. There are additional cardiac conditions that require preoperative planning. Patients with permanent pacemaker or an automatic implantable cardioverter-defibrillator may need evaluation and device interrogation. The management of these devices should be individualized based on patients' underlying rhythm and function. Management of anticoagulated patients is controversial. The withdrawal of these agents prematurely is a major risk for stent thrombosis, especially for drug-eluting stents.[19,21] However, the continuation of these agents may significantly increase the risk of bleeding. Blood loss should be closely monitored and replaced, especially in the patient population at high risk. A multidisciplinary consensus approach should be adopted for the management of these challenging patients.[7,21,22]

Pulmonary Consideration in Patients with Hip Fracture and Risk Stratification

Pulmonary complications are the second most frequent adverse medical events, affecting 4% of all patients with hip fracture with 3% of patients experiencing severe complications.[3] It not only prolongs the length of hospitalization but also is related to perioperative mortality and morbidity.[25,26]

Risk factors for respiratory failure may be categorized from a mechanistic standpoint into the following groups.

(1) Risks related to the increased demand on oxygen consumption and impaired oxygen supply during the perioperative period. Acute stress response to the surgery, pain related to the fracture and surgical insult, systemic inflammatory response to surgery, fever, or sepsis could also lead to an elevated metabolic state and increase oxygen demand.[6] Although the oxygen demand is increased during the perioperative period, the oxygen supply might not be able to match it among this aged and complicated patient population. Atelectasis could shift the ventilation-perfusion mismatch and result in hypoxia.[27] Sedatives, especially opioid analgesics, could depress respiratory effort and thus impair oxygenation and ventilation.

(2) Risks related to airway protection. General anesthesia and narcotics could impair effective cough and epithelium clearance.[28] Patients with changes in mental status are also at increased risk of aspiration pneumonia and respiratory failure.

Although pulmonary complications are detrimental, the goal of risk stratification is relatively straightforward.[29] First, one needs to establish the degree of risk based on patient comorbidities and surgical risks. Clinical evaluation and spirometry can collect essential information for decision making. Patients with room air oxygen saturation less than 90%, forced expiratory volume in 1 second less than 47%, forced vital capacity less than 1.7 L, and peak expiratory flow rate less than 82 L/min might experience difficulty with ventilation and oxygenation.[30,31] Although these patients may still proceed to surgery, close respiratory monitoring, pulmonary toileting, and even continuous ventilatory support might be needed. Second, providers should aim for early intervention to optimize the patient's condition preoperatively, along with continuous management to reduce the perioperative risks. It might be important to seek expertise from multiple disciplines early for patients with hip fracture at high risk for pulmonary complication. These experts should include an anesthesiologist, pulmonologist, and intensivist.[32]

Potential pulmonary complications include pneumonia, atelectasis, pulmonary embolism, exacerbation of a chronic lung condition, acute respiratory distress syndrome, or respiratory failure.[33] There are many patient-related risk factors, such as advanced age, impaired sensorium, function dependency, congestive heart failure (CHF), chronic obstructive pulmonary disease (COPD), obstructive sleep apnea (OSA), ascites, albumin less than 35 g/L, creatinine greater than 1.5 mg/dL, or blood urea nitrogen greater than 21 mg/dL.[32,34–36] The pulmonary risk index has been validated to predict pneumonia and respiratory failure after noncardiac surgery.[32,35,36] This index is a calculated point value with different weight on multiple risk factors, such as American Society of Anesthesiologists (ASA) status, type of surgery, age, functional status, general anesthesia, emergency surgery, and existing medical conditions (COPD, CHF, history of cerebrovascular accident, current smoker, and so forth.).[35,36] Functional dependency is an important predictor of postoperative pulmonary complication (odds ratio 2.51).[34]

In addition there are also surgical risk factors, including general anesthesia, use of long-acting neuromuscular blockade, emergency surgery, and prolonged operation time.[6,32,35,36] Although some of the surgical risk factors may be unavoidable, a systemic approach should be used to minimize the exposure of these surgical risk factors.

COPD is associated with increased risks of pulmonary complication.[37–40] However, surgery is not contraindicated even in patients with severe COPD.[41] The goal of perioperative management on patients with severe COPD is to optimize the disease and minimize the risks of pulmonary complications.[42] The challenge for the managing physician is to optimize the management of COPD efficiently and effectively within a short period of time. It might be beneficial to involve a pulmonologist and a respiratory therapist early in the process. The drugs of choices are bronchodilators such as anticholinergic agents and/or β2-agonists,[43,44] while suspected bacterial pneumonia should be treated with antibiotics as per institutional guidelines.[45]

Asthma per se is not a risk factor for pulmonary complications among surgical patients.[46] However, uncontrolled asthma, such as frequent rescue inhaler use and recent asthma symptoms, have been associated with a higher risk of pulmonary complications.[46] Intense preoperative treatment with anticholinergic agents and/or β2-agonists should be indicated to optimize the patient's condition.[47] Systematic steroids have been used in managing poorly controlled asthma patients preoperatively,[48] although there are concerns about risks of infection and delayed wound healing.[49,50]

OSA is associated with a higher incidence of pulmonary complications among patients undergoing major orthopedic surgery.[51] The major concerns among OSA patients are 2-fold. First, OSA patients tend to have higher incidence of difficult airway and right-side–dominant CHF.[38] Second, anesthesia and analgesia would further hinder the hypoxia and hypercarbia response of these already impaired OSA patients.[52] The ASA guideline recommends that adequate treatment such as continuous positive airway pressure (CPAP) or other appliances should be provided during the perioperative period.[53] It is also important to evaluate suspected OSA patients and thus implement prophylaxis treatment. The STOP questionnaire is a simple validated tool used to screen patients for OSA.[54]

Existing pneumonia or recent change of sputum production is associated with postoperative pulmonary complications. Antibiotic treatment should be initiated and continued. However, viral infection in the upper respiratory airway was not associated with an increased risk of pulmonary complications.[46] Even for patients with acute pneumonia, the condition may or may not improve, especially with existing hip fracture and immobility. Surgical fixation of the hip fracture might be still desirable in the setting of inadequate pulmonary reserve.[55]

Other chronic respiratory findings, such as cough, dyspnea, wheezing, or rales, should initiate further evaluation of potential underlying cardiopulmonary status. A detailed history and physical examination would be sufficient to identify patients for further workups. Although cardiac etiology could compromise the evaluation, patients with an unexplained or worsening respiratory condition need to be evaluated by spirometry preoperatively.[56] The bronchodilator response, either restrictive or obstructive, is especially valuable in guiding the differential diagnosis. Subsequently it could also guide therapeutic intervention to optimize the pulmonary condition.[57] Nonetheless, because most patients with hip fracture are seniors with limited functional capacity, it is more challenging to distinguish between cardiac and pulmonary causes. Judicious use of echocardiography in addition to spirometry can provide important information for differential diagnosis and perioperative management. Although many lung diseases are major concerns during the perioperative period, the evidence of increased risk of pulmonary complications is lacking among patients with hip fracture.[34] Balanced surgical decisions and management are recommended.

Although many individual risk factors have been identified, ASA classification is a reliable and relatively simple predictor of postoperative pulmonary complications among patients undergoing noncardiothoracic surgery.[58] Patients in ASA class 2 or higher have a higher risk of pulmonary complications (odds ratio 4.87).[59] ASA classification has also been confirmed to be a convenient way to stratify the pulmonary risk of patients with hip fracture.[59]

In consideration of all these risk factors, the authors propose a simplified algorithm to guide the management of patients with hip fracture, assuming the hip fracture is a closed fracture and thus semi-urgent in nature (**Fig. 2**).

Step 1. Does the patient have an active pulmonary condition? The surgery should proceed if there is no active pulmonary condition or when the pulmonary condition is stable. However, some patients warrant further workup, including those with existing pneumonia, severe COPD with oxygen requirement, or symptomatic OSA. The workup may include laboratory and imaging studies, pulmonary function tests, sleep study, and pulmonology consult.

Step 2. Is there any opportunity to stabilize or improve the patient's baseline pulmonary condition? For example, patients with decompensated COPD should be managed collectively by a pulmonologist, respiratory therapist, intensivist, and anesthesiologist. The decision of whether and when surgery should proceed needs to be individualized for each patient, but should be a team decision with the patient's understanding and agreement.

Risk of Venous Thromboembolism

Patients with hip fractures are at higher risk of developing venous thromboembolism (VTE) and potential detrimental pulmonary embolism. Thromboprophylaxis treatment has been recommended by the American College of Chest Physicians, and implemented in clinical practice extensively.[60] However, it is estimated that 9% of patients will still develop VTE even with aggressive thromboprophylaxis treatment.[61] Thromboprophylaxis treatment is commonly started before the surgery, owing to the high risk of deep vein thrombosis before the planned surgical time.[62] In contrast, however, comparable protection with postsurgical thromboprophylaxis has been reported.[63] In addition, initiating thromboprophylaxis after surgery eliminates its potential for intraoperative bleeding risk, and the concern about associated risks with neuraxial anesthesia and peripheral nerve blocks.

Pharmacologic treatment options include unfractionated heparin, low molecular weight heparin, warfarin, and, in some cases, aspirin. The practice has various institutional and physician variation.[64,65] For patients with contraindications to anticoagulation, such as bleeding disorder or high bleeding risk, pneumatic sequential leg compression should be applied nonetheless.[66]

Delirium

Delirium is common among hospitalized patients, especially senior patients with pre-existing cognitive impairment.[67] Delirium can affect 35% to 65% of patients with hip fracture and is an independent risk factor for worse surgical outcome.[59,68] The current appreciation of the mechanism of delirium is a combination of predisposing and precipitating factors, while the management goal is prevention.[69] Although anesthesia and analgesia are mandatory for the management of patients with hip fracture, anesthesia and analgesia are also discredited for delirium. Nonetheless, it is important to emphasize risk-factor modification among patients with hip fracture to mitigate precipitating factors, including measures such as adequate postoperative pain control and geriatrics consultation.[68–70] A prophylactic low dose of haloperidol was also suggested to decrease the severity and duration of delirium.[70,71]

Other Preoperative Medical Considerations

Preoperative tests such as chest radiography, spirometry, and echocardiography should not be ordered as a routine for preoperative workup. The results of these tests have little impact on the decision making and perioperative management for the

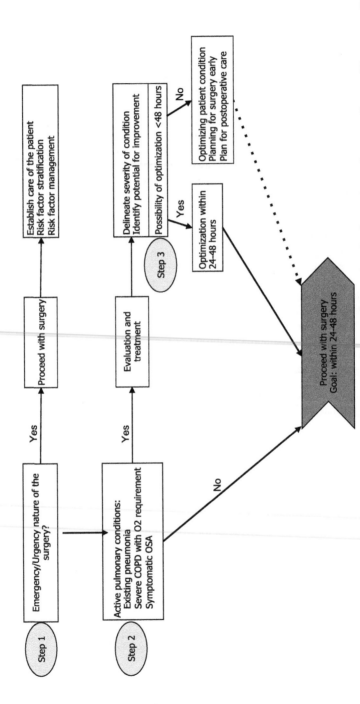

Fig. 2. Pulmonary evaluation and care algorithm for patients with hip fracture. COPD, chronic obstructive pulmonary disease; O2, oxygen; OSA, obstructive sleep apnea.

general patient population with hip fracture.[34] Chest radiography is expected to alter the management plan in a very small percentage of patients, and is therefore not recommended as a routine test.[72,73] However, a chest radiograph should be considered for patients with unexplained or unstable respiratory symptoms or suspected lower respiratory tract infection.[55] A similar recommendation also applies to spirometry. Spirometry can be very informative in providing baseline information on pulmonary function, and to provide information on the current status of COPD or asthma, and is recommended for patients with active respiratory symptoms.[56]

Recommendation

Surgical treatment of hip fracture should be performed nonemergently and within 24 to 48 hours. The goal of preoperative management is to review the medical condition, delineate the severity of disease, and, most importantly, determine whether improvement in the medical condition is achieved in a timely manner to improve the patient's outcome. Although many institutions still seek medical clearance mainly for medicolegal reasons, it might delay the surgical treatment and inadvertently expose patients to worse outcomes. The decision to proceed should be a team decision with patient's or caregiver's approval (**Fig. 3**).

Step 1. Risk assessment of the patient based on medical condition. The essential question is whether improvement in the medical condition can be achieved in a timely manner. Surgery should proceed with minimal preoperative preparation if the patient has minimal perioperative risk. However, the surgeon should seek early consultation for other specialties should the patient have moderate coexisting conditions while stable. The purpose of consultation is to coordinate multidisciplinary treatment and planning throughout the preoperative, intraoperative, and postoperative periods.

Step 2. Determine whether optimization of medical condition can be achieved in a timely manner for patients with an unstable severe medical condition. Although surgical risk is detrimental, the delay in surgical treatment would also hinder the chance of a patient's quality of recovery. There are only limited conditions that might justify delaying surgical repair of a hip fracture, such as acute renal injury, severe electrolyte abnormality (such as potassium <2.8 or >6.0 mmol/L), uncontrolled diabetes with risks or signs of acidosis or even coma, and severe coagulopathy.[6] The medical decision regarding treatment should be individualized according to the fundamental principle of no harm to the patient and respecting the patient's wishes.

INTRAOPERATIVE CONSIDERATIONS
Surgical Considerations

The primary goal of surgical treatment is safe and effective stabilization of the injury site to allow the recovery of all organ systems, including the remobilization of the musculoskeletal system. Definitive surgery not only allows the long-term functional recovery process but also helps medical management by allowing improved pulmonary toilet/function, decreased cardiac sympathetic load mitigating pain from an unstable fracture, and thereby the return of physical self-autonomy to the patient.[74,75]

At baseline, the perioperative team should understand several important elements of the patient's fracture itself. The term "hip fracture" refers classically to 2 injuries: the intracapsular femoral neck fracture and intertrochanteric (between the greater and lesser trochanters) fracture. Some also consider the "subtroch," or subtrochanteric fracture, a hip fracture. Although all the related surgeries are considered moderately invasive, they differ somewhat from the surgical point of view.

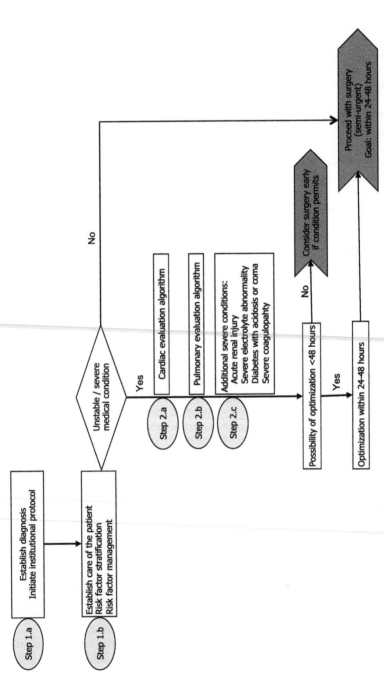

Fig. 3. Institutional care algorithm for patients with hip fracture. See **Fig. 1** for details on step 2.a (cardiac evaluation and care algorithm). See **Fig. 2** for details on step 2.b (pulmonary evaluation and care algorithm).

Most intertrochanteric hip (and subtrochanteric) fractures are treated with minimally invasive reduction and fixation using a "nail" (interlocking rod) or a sliding hip screw (plate-and-screw device). The invasiveness here is not determined by the size of the incision (though they are typically small) but more from the fact that the fracture site is not formally exposed, thus allowing for decreased physiologic insult to the surrounding tissue and blood loss to the patient as a result of surgery. Aside from the reaming (about midway through procedure used for long nails), when there will be a sympathetic load from endosteal disruption and the potential for fatty pulmonary emboli, the procedure should not be stressful for the patient, surgeon, or anesthesia provider. The placement of sliding hip screws and short nails should be even less of a physiologic stress or burden on the patient. The length and invasiveness of most of these procedures, and the supine position of the patient, should allow for many anesthetic options including neuraxial methods.

The other major category is femoral neck fractures. These patients demographically tend to be slightly older and represent about one-half of hip fractures in the elderly. The treatment decisions for these hip fractures tend to diverge more than for intertrochanteric fractures. The first decision is between fixation and replacement. Fixation potentially preserves native anatomy but overall has lower functional results than replacement. In the perioperative period, the implications are 2-fold. Closed reduction and percutaneous or limited open fixation represents a type of procedure (time, blood loss, stress) similar to that described above. Formal open reduction and fixation, on the other hand, could represent a much bigger surgery and is typically reserved for those physiologically younger. The replacement options for fracture fixation do not differ much from those done for arthritis. These procedures require formal open exposure (even when minimally invasive), excision of the unstable fracture, and replacement with a femoral component with (total arthroplasty) or without (hemi-arthroplasty) an acetabular component. These surgeries can also typically be performed within the time constraints of intrathecal anesthetic, but represent greater physiologic stress (larger incision, more dissection, resection, blood loss) than for less invasive fixation.

Fixation or replacement is performed with the goal of allowing weight bearing as tolerated after surgery in almost all cases. Fixation typically will have no positional restrictions, whereas many replacement surgeries will have specific restrictions on range of motion. Postoperative mobilization will need to be performed with this in mind. Chemoprophylaxis for VTE should also be administered with consideration of bleeding and wound risk. As one might expect, wound and bleeding concerns are decreased with the less invasive procedures (eg, nailing, closed reduction with percutaneous fixation).

The Choice of Anesthesia

It has long been debated about which anesthesia technique is better: general anesthesia (GA) or spinal/epidural anesthesia (SEA). Many clinical trials have attempted to compare SEA and GA in hip fracture surgery, with inconclusive results, mainly because of the sample size,[76–80] while some have reported conflicting results.[4,81] Neuman and colleagues[82] studied a New York State inpatient database with 18,158 patients, and found that SEA is associated with lower odds of mortality and pulmonary complications. However, White and colleagues[83] conducted an observational study on the United Kingdom National Hip Fracture Database with 65,535 patients, and concluded that there was no difference in 30-day mortality between GA and SEA. Meta-analysis on mortality and morbidity with SEA versus GA indicated that SEA is not inferior to GA.[84–86] SEA is thus generally recommended for most patients, considering there is no contraindication.

POSTOPERATIVE CARE

Systematic planning of postoperative care of patients with hip fracture should be initiated preoperatively. The primary care team (eg, intensivist, pulmonologist, cardiologist) should align necessary support. The primary goal of the postoperative period is to provide hemodynamic stabilization, continue aggressive pulmonary treatment (such as incentive spirometry, deep-breathing exercises, and chest physical therapy), minimize risk factors and incidence of delirium, provide adequate analgesia, and allow for safe and expedient mobilization.[87]

INSTITUTIONAL GUIDELINES

It is general practice that each institution develops a consensus or guideline for the management of patients with hip fracture to avoid systematic errors that might delay the necessary care of patients with hip fracture and to improve efficiency. Emergency room physicians are usually the frontline medical specialists to first recognize and initiate the institutional protocol. Early intervention with necessary specialists can arrest further deterioration, achieve earlier optimization of condition, and acquire quick surgical treatment. Invariably such guidelines may allow deviations regarding patients' specific situations. Input from all specialties should be summoned to meet the best interests of patients.

REFERENCES

1. Kannus P, Parkkari J, Sievanen H, et al. Epidemiology of hip fractures. Bone 1996;18:57S–63S.
2. Roche JJ, Wenn RT, Sahota O, et al. Effect of comorbidities and postoperative complications on mortality after hip fracture in elderly people: prospective observational cohort study. BMJ 2005;331:1374.
3. Lawrence VA, Hilsenbeck SG, Noveck H, et al. Medical complications and outcomes after hip fracture repair. Arch Intern Med 2002;162:2053–7.
4. Radcliff TA, Henderson WG, Stoner TJ, et al. Patient risk factors, operative care, and outcomes among older community-dwelling male veterans with hip fracture. J Bone Joint Surg Am 2008;90:34–42.
5. Shiga T, Wajima Z, Ohe Y. Is operative delay associated with increased mortality of hip fracture patients? Systematic review, meta-analysis, and meta-regression. Can J Anaesth 2008;55:146–54.
6. Wong GT, Sun NC. Providing perioperative care for patients with hip fractures. Osteoporos Int 2010;21:S547–53.
7. Fleisher LA, Fleischmann KE, Auerbach AD, et al. 2014 ACC/AHA Guideline on Perioperative Cardiovascular Evaluation and Management of Patients Undergoing Noncardiac Surgery: Executive Summary: A Report of the American College of Cardiology/American Heart Association Task Force on Practice Guidelines. Circulation 2014. [Epub ahead of print].
8. Fleisher LA, Beckman JA, Brown KA, et al. ACC/AHA 2007 guidelines on perioperative cardiovascular evaluation and care for noncardiac surgery: executive summary: a report of the American College of Cardiology/American Heart Association Task Force on Practice Guidelines (Writing Committee to Revise the 2002 Guidelines on Perioperative Cardiovascular Evaluation for Noncardiac Surgery): developed in Collaboration with the American Society of Echocardiography, American Society of Nuclear Cardiology, Heart Rhythm Society, Society of Cardiovascular Anesthesiologists, Society for Cardiovascular Angiography and

Interventions, Society for Vascular Medicine and Biology, and Society for Vascular Surgery. Circulation 2007;116:1971–96.

9. Fleisher LA, Beckman JA, Brown KA, et al. ACC/AHA 2007 guidelines on perioperative cardiovascular evaluation and care for noncardiac surgery: a report of the American College of Cardiology/American Heart Association Task Force on Practice Guidelines (Writing Committee to Revise the 2002 Guidelines on Perioperative Cardiovascular Evaluation for Noncardiac Surgery): developed in collaboration with the American Society of Echocardiography, American Society of Nuclear Cardiology, Heart Rhythm Society, Society of Cardiovascular Anesthesiologists, Society for Cardiovascular Angiography and Interventions, Society for Vascular Medicine and Biology, and Society for Vascular Surgery. Circulation 2007;116:e418–99.

10. Komarasamy B, Forster MC, Esler CN, et al. Mortality following hip fracture surgery in patients with recent myocardial infarction. Ann R Coll Surg Engl 2007;89:521–5.

11. Carbone L, Buzkova P, Fink HA, et al. Hip fractures and heart failure: findings from the Cardiovascular Health Study. Eur Heart J 2010;31:77–84.

12. Lee TH, Marcantonio ER, Mangione CM, et al. Derivation and prospective validation of a simple index for prediction of cardiac risk of major noncardiac surgery. Circulation 1999;100:1043–9.

13. Lindroos M, Kupari M, Heikkila J, et al. Prevalence of aortic valve abnormalities in the elderly: an echocardiographic study of a random population sample. J Am Coll Cardiol 1993;21:1220–5.

14. Stewart BF, Siscovick D, Lind BK, et al. Clinical factors associated with calcific aortic valve disease. Cardiovascular Health Study. J Am Coll Cardiol 1997;29:630–4.

15. Chambers J. Aortic stenosis. BMJ 2005;330:801–2.

16. Detsky AS, Abrams HB, Forbath N, et al. Cardiac assessment for patients undergoing noncardiac surgery. A multifactorial clinical risk index. Arch Intern Med 1986;146:2131–4.

17. Goldman L, Caldera DL, Nussbaum SR, et al. Multifactorial index of cardiac risk in noncardiac surgical procedures. N Engl J Med 1977;297:845–50.

18. McBrien ME, Heyburn G, Stevenson M, et al. Previously undiagnosed aortic stenosis revealed by auscultation in the hip fracture population—echocardiographic findings, management and outcome. Anaesthesia 2009;64:863–70.

19. Adunsky A, Kaplan A, Arad M, et al. Aortic stenosis in elderly hip fractured patients. Arch Gerontol Geriatr 2008;46:401–8.

20. Siu CW, Sun NC, Lau TW, et al. Preoperative cardiac risk assessment in geriatric patients with hip fractures: an orthopedic surgeons' perspective. Osteoporos Int 2010;21:S587–91.

21. Bartels C, Bechtel JF, Hossmann V, et al. Cardiac risk stratification for high-risk vascular surgery. Circulation 1997;95:2473–5.

22. Myers J, Do D, Herbert W, et al. A nomogram to predict exercise capacity from a specific activity questionnaire and clinical data. Am J Cardiol 1994;73:591–6.

23. Nelson CL, Herndon JE, Mark DB, et al. Relation of clinical and angiographic factors to functional capacity as measured by the Duke Activity Status Index. Am J Cardiol 1991;68:973–5.

24. Older P, Hall A, Hader R. Cardiopulmonary exercise testing as a screening test for perioperative management of major surgery in the elderly. Chest 1999;116:355–62.

25. Liu LL, Leung JM. Predicting adverse postoperative outcomes in patients aged 80 years or older. J Am Geriatr Soc 2000;48:405–12.
26. Smetana GW. Preoperative pulmonary evaluation. N Engl J Med 1999;340:937–44.
27. Magnusson L, Spahn DR. New concepts of atelectasis during general anaesthesia. Br J Anaesth 2003;91:61–72.
28. Gamsu G, Singer MM, Vincent HH, et al. Postoperative impairment of mucous transport in the lung. Am Rev Respir Dis 1976;114:673–9.
29. Smetana GW. Preoperative pulmonary assessment of the older adult. Clin Geriatr Med 2003;19:35–55.
30. Smina M, Salam A, Khamiees M, et al. Cough peak flows and extubation outcomes. Chest 2003;124:262–8.
31. Montes de Oca M, Celli BR. Mouth occlusion pressure, CO_2 response and hypercapnia in severe chronic obstructive pulmonary disease. Eur Respir J 1998;12:666–71.
32. Arozullah AM, Daley J, Henderson WG, et al. Multifactorial risk index for predicting postoperative respiratory failure in men after major noncardiac surgery. The National Veterans Administration Surgical Quality Improvement Program. Ann Surg 2000;232:242–53.
33. Swenson E. Preoperative pulmonary evaluation. In: Albert RK, Spiro S, Jett J, editors. Clinical respiratory medicine. 2nd edition. Philadelphia: Elsevier Science; 2004. p. 229–34.
34. Qaseem A, Snow V, Fitterman N, et al. Risk assessment for and strategies to reduce perioperative pulmonary complications for patients undergoing noncardiothoracic surgery: a guideline from the American College of Physicians. Ann Intern Med 2006;144:575–80.
35. Arozullah AM, Khuri SF, Henderson WG, et al. Development and validation of a multifactorial risk index for predicting postoperative pneumonia after major noncardiac surgery. Ann Intern Med 2001;135:847–57.
36. Johnson RG, Arozullah AM, Neumayer L, et al. Multivariable predictors of postoperative respiratory failure after general and vascular surgery: results from the patient safety in surgery study. J Am Coll Surg 2007;204:1188–98.
37. Warner DO, Warner MA, Offord KP, et al. Airway obstruction and perioperative complications in smokers undergoing abdominal surgery. Anesthesiology 1999;90:372–9.
38. McAlister FA, Khan NA, Straus SE, et al. Accuracy of the preoperative assessment in predicting pulmonary risk after nonthoracic surgery. Am J Respir Crit Care Med 2003;167:741–4.
39. Fisher BW, Majumdar SR, McAlister FA. Predicting pulmonary complications after nonthoracic surgery: a systematic review of blinded studies. Am J Med 2002;112:219–25.
40. Gass GD, Olsen GN. Preoperative pulmonary function testing to predict postoperative morbidity and mortality. Chest 1986;89:127–35.
41. Kroenke K, Lawrence VA, Theroux JF, et al. Operative risk in patients with severe obstructive pulmonary disease. Arch Intern Med 1992;152:967–71.
42. Alifano M, Cuvelier A, Delage A, et al. Treatment of COPD: from pharmacological to instrumental therapies. Eur Respir Rev 2010;19:7–23.
43. McCrory DC, Brown CD. Anti-cholinergic bronchodilators versus beta2-sympathomimetic agents for acute exacerbations of chronic obstructive pulmonary disease. Cochrane Database Syst Rev 2002;(4):CD003900.
44. Johnson M, Rennard S. Alternative mechanisms for long-acting beta(2)-adrenergic agonists in COPD. Chest 2001;120:258–70.

45. Wilson R, Jones P, Schaberg T, et al. Antibiotic treatment and factors influencing short and long term outcomes of acute exacerbations of chronic bronchitis. Thorax 2006;61:337–42.
46. Warner DO, Warner MA, Barnes RD, et al. Perioperative respiratory complications in patients with asthma. Anesthesiology 1996;85:460–7.
47. Bateman ED, Hurd SS, Barnes PJ, et al. Global strategy for asthma management and prevention: GINA executive summary. Eur Respir J 2008;31:143–78.
48. Silvanus MT, Groeben H, Peters J. Corticosteroids and inhaled salbutamol in patients with reversible airway obstruction markedly decrease the incidence of bronchospasm after tracheal intubation. Anesthesiology 2004;100:1052–7.
49. Pien LC, Grammer LC, Patterson R. Minimal complications in a surgical population with severe asthma receiving prophylactic corticosteroids. J Allergy Clin Immunol 1988;82:696–700.
50. Kabalin CS, Yarnold PR, Grammer LC. Low complication rate of corticosteroid-treated asthmatics undergoing surgical procedures. Arch Intern Med 1995;155: 1379–84.
51. Gupta RM, Parvizi J, Hanssen AD, et al. Postoperative complications in patients with obstructive sleep apnea syndrome undergoing hip or knee replacement: a case-control study. Mayo Clin Proc 2001;76:897–905.
52. Rock P, Passannante A. Preoperative assessment: pulmonary. Anesthesiol Clin North America 2004;22:77–91.
53. Gross JB, Bachenberg KL, Benumof JL, et al. Practice guidelines for the perioperative management of patients with obstructive sleep apnea: a report by the American Society of Anesthesiologists Task Force on perioperative management of patients with obstructive sleep apnea. Anesthesiology 2006;104:1081–93 [quiz: 1117–8].
54. Chung F, Yegneswaran B, Liao P, et al. STOP questionnaire: a tool to screen patients for obstructive sleep apnea. Anesthesiology 2008;108:812–21.
55. Lo IL, Siu CW, Tse HF, et al. Pre-operative pulmonary assessment for patients with hip fracture. Osteoporos Int 2010;21:S579–86.
56. Preoperative pulmonary function testing. American College of Physicians. Ann Intern Med 1990;112:793–4.
57. Pellegrino R, Viegi G, Brusasco V, et al. Interpretative strategies for lung function tests. Eur Respir J 2005;26:948–68.
58. Owens WD, Felts JA, Spitznagel EL Jr. ASA physical status classifications: a study of consistency of ratings. Anesthesiology 1978;49:239–43.
59. Smetana GW, Lawrence VA, Cornell JE. Preoperative pulmonary risk stratification for noncardiothoracic surgery: systematic review for the American College of Physicians. Ann Intern Med 2006;144:581–95.
60. Geerts WH, Bergqvist D, Pineo GF, et al. Prevention of venous thromboembolism: American College of Chest Physicians evidence-based clinical practice guidelines (8th edition). Chest 2008;133:381S–453S.
61. Schiff RL, Kahn SR, Shrier I, et al. Identifying orthopedic patients at high risk for venous thromboembolism despite thromboprophylaxis. Chest 2005;128: 3364–71.
62. Morrison RS, Chassin MR, Siu AL. The medical consultant's role in caring for patients with hip fracture. Ann Intern Med 1998;128:1010–20.
63. Hull RD, Pineo GF, Francis C, et al. Low-molecular-weight heparin prophylaxis using dalteparin in close proximity to surgery vs warfarin in hip arthroplasty patients: a double-blind, randomized comparison. The North American Fragmin Trial Investigators. Arch Intern Med 2000;160:2199–207.

64. Francis CW. Prevention of VTE in patients having major orthopedic surgery. J Thromb Thrombolysis 2013;35:359–67.
65. Tufano A, Coppola A, Cerbone AM, et al. Preventing postsurgical venous thromboembolism: pharmacological approaches. Semin Thromb Hemost 2011;37: 252–66.
66. Handoll HH, Farrar MJ, McBirnie J, et al. Heparin, low molecular weight heparin and physical methods for preventing deep vein thrombosis and pulmonary embolism following surgery for hip fractures. Cochrane Database Syst Rev 2002;(4):CD000305.
67. Trzepacz PT. Delirium. Advances in diagnosis, pathophysiology, and treatment. Psychiatr Clin North Am 1996;19:429–48.
68. Marcantonio ER, Flacker JM, Wright RJ, et al. Reducing delirium after hip fracture: a randomized trial. J Am Geriatr Soc 2001;49:516–22.
69. Sieber FE. Postoperative delirium in the elderly surgical patient. Anesthesiol Clin 2009;27:451–64 table of contents.
70. Siddiqi N, Stockdale R, Britton AM, et al. Interventions for preventing delirium in hospitalised patients. Cochrane Database Syst Rev 2007;(2):CD005563.
71. Kalisvaart KJ, de Jonghe JF, Bogaards MJ, et al. Haloperidol prophylaxis for elderly hip-surgery patients at risk for delirium: a randomized placebo-controlled study. J Am Geriatr Soc 2005;53:1658–66.
72. Joo HS, Wong J, Naik VN, et al. The value of screening preoperative chest x-rays: a systematic review. Can J Anaesth 2005;52:568–74.
73. Archer C, Levy AR, McGregor M. Value of routine preoperative chest x-rays: a meta-analysis. Can J Anaesth 1993;40:1022–7.
74. Kaplan K, Miyamoto R, Levine BR, et al. Surgical management of hip fractures: an evidence-based review of the literature. II: intertrochanteric fractures. J Am Acad Orthop Surg 2008;16:665–73.
75. Miyamoto RG, Kaplan KM, Levine BR, et al. Surgical management of hip fractures: an evidence-based review of the literature. I: femoral neck fractures. J Am Acad Orthop Surg 2008;16:596–607.
76. Berggren D, Gustafson Y, Eriksson B, et al. Postoperative confusion after anesthesia in elderly patients with femoral neck fractures. Anesth Analg 1987;66: 497–504.
77. Davis FM, Laurenson VG. Spinal anaesthesia or general anaesthesia for emergency hip surgery in elderly patients. Anaesth Intensive Care 1981;9: 352–8.
78. Juelsgaard P, Sand NP, Felsby S, et al. Perioperative myocardial ischaemia in patients undergoing surgery for fractured hip randomized to incremental spinal, single-dose spinal or general anaesthesia. Eur J Anaesthesiol 1998;15: 656–63.
79. Racle JP, Benkhadra A, Poy JY, et al. Comparative study of general and spinal anesthesia in elderly women in hip surgery. Ann Fr Anesth Reanim 1986;5:24–30 [in French].
80. Valentin N, Lomholt B, Jensen JS, et al. Spinal or general anaesthesia for surgery of the fractured hip? A prospective study of mortality in 578 patients. Br J Anaesth 1986;58:284–91.
81. O'Hara DA, Duff A, Berlin JA, et al. The effect of anesthetic technique on postoperative outcomes in hip fracture repair. Anesthesiology 2000;92:947–57.
82. Neuman MD, Silber JH, Elkassabany NM, et al. Comparative effectiveness of regional versus general anesthesia for hip fracture surgery in adults. Anesthesiology 2012;117:72–92.

83. White SM, Moppett IK, Griffiths R. Outcome by mode of anaesthesia for hip fracture surgery. An observational audit of 65 535 patients in a national dataset. Anaesthesia 2014;69:224–30.

84. Beaupre LA, Jones CA, Saunders LD, et al. Best practices for elderly hip fracture patients. A systematic overview of the evidence. J Gen Intern Med 2005;20: 1019–25.

85. Rodgers A, Walker N, Schug S, et al. Reduction of postoperative mortality and morbidity with epidural or spinal anaesthesia: results from overview of randomised trials. BMJ 2000;321:1493.

86. Parker MJ, Handoll HH, Griffiths R. Anaesthesia for hip fracture surgery in adults. Cochrane Database Syst Rev 2004;(4):CD000521.

87. Mak JC, Cameron ID, March LM. Evidence-based guidelines for the management of hip fractures in older persons: an update. Med J Aust 2010; 192:37–41.

Regional Anesthesia-Analgesia

Relationship to Cancer Recurrence and Infection

Benjamin A. Vaghari, MD, Omar I. Ahmed, MD,
Christopher L. Wu, MD*

KEYWORDS

- Regional anesthesia • Epidural • Cancer • Infection

KEY POINTS

- Perioperative immune function is important for the development of cancer recurrence and surgical site infection.
- Use of regional anesthesia-analgesia (with a local anesthetic-based regimen) as part of a multidisciplinary approach may attenuate perioperative immunosuppression and provide the physiologic basis for decreasing cancer recurrence and surgical site infection.
- Currently available data examining the relationship between regional anesthesia-analgesia and decreasing cancer recurrence or surgical site infection do not provide any definitive answers due in part to the heterogeneous nature of cancer studied and the limited (methodologic) nature of the studies currently published.
- Although most data are published on nonorthopedic surgical patients, the general principles are similar and can be applied to orthopedic surgical patients.

INTRODUCTION

Patients undergoing surgical procedures will exhibit a transient period of immunosuppression that may provide the permissive circumstances for cancer recurrence or surgical site infections (SSIs). Use of regional anesthesia-analgesia, especially when using a local anesthetic-based regimen, can preserve perioperative immune function and provide the physiologic basis for decreased cancer recurrence and SSI, especially when used as part of a multidisciplinary approach. Although there is little direct

No disclosures.
Department of Anesthesiology and Critical Care Medicine, Johns Hopkins University School of Medicine, 1800 Orleans Street, Baltimore, MD 21287, USA
* Corresponding author. Johns Hopkins University, Zayed 8-120, 1800 Orleans Street, Baltimore, MD 21287.
E-mail address: chwu@jhmi.edu

anesthesiology.theclinics.com

evidence or data investigating orthopedic patients, the basic concepts of the immune system and cancer recurrence/infection are reviewed, which are applicable to all patients, including those undergoing orthopedic procedures, and the available peer-reviewed publications examining the relationship between regional anesthesia-analgesia and these outcomes.

THE IMMUNE SYSTEM AND CANCER

The hypothesis that the immune system is responsible for cancer elimination and suppression is not new.[1] Individuals with suppressed immune systems, such as those with human immunodeficiency virus or requiring immunosuppressive agents after organ transplantation, show increased risks of cancer development.[2–4] A properly functioning immune system is vital in reducing cancer occurrence for the individual. However, the interplay between the immune system and cancer cells is complex and has led to the development of the theory of "immunoediting."

The concept of immunoediting involves 3 phases.[1] The first phase is elimination. This elimination phase entails cells of the innate and adaptive immune system seeking out and eliminating cancer cells. Evidence suggests that individuals with increased natural cytotoxic activity have decreased cancer risk.[5] However, despite this effort at tumor cell control, elimination is not always successful (ie, cancer cells are heterogeneous, and some cancer cells are more susceptible to being killed than others, similar to the concept of antibiotic resistance), leading to the second "equilibrium" phase.[1] In the equilibrium phase, the cancer cells are held in check by the immune system and cancer cells that display decreased immunogenicity are selected, subsequently leading to the third phase of "escape." In this phase, the cancer cells that are more successful at escaping the immune system can result in metastatic tumors.[1]

SURGICAL STRESS LEADS TO IMMUNOSUPPRESSION VIA STRESS RESPONSE

Once tumors are present, surgical excision is often offered as a major treatment option. However, surgery is not often curative because minimal residual disease, either at the tumor margins or at micrometastases at distant sites, can be present. Surgery may actually increase growth in previously unrecognized micrometastases and create an environment that promotes further metastatic spread.[6] As these remaining cancer cells continue to divide, the cellular immune response is often weakened within hours of surgery and lasts for days.[7] This temporary immunosuppression is a result of the neuroendocrine-mediated and cytokine-mediated stress response to surgery. As cellular immunity (an important component of which includes natural killer cells) decreases, cancer morbidity then increases.[8,9] Greater surgical trauma leads to greater suppression of the cellular immune system.[7] In a mouse model, increasing surgical stress leads to a direct increase in metastases.[10] Laparoscopy, which is less invasive than open resection of colorectal cancer, has been shown to be associated with both increased disease-free time and increased time to recurrence.[11] Thus, as surgical stress decreases the immune response, a window period is created that appears to give cancer cells an opportunity to spread. Although surgical stress is an important component, pain can also play a role in immunomodulation.

Pain, much like surgery, can incite the stress response and lead to immunosuppression. Acute pain has been shown to decrease cellular immunity and potentially lead to tumor promotion.[12] How that pain is managed in the perioperative period can have important implications in mediating the stress response, the resulting immunomodulation, and cancer growth.

OPIOIDS AND THE IMMUNE SYSTEM

Opioid medications, routinely used as the mainstay of postsurgical analgesia, are themselves not benign and can exert effects on the immune system. Morphine has been shown to inhibit natural killer cell cytotoxicity in healthy volunteers.[13] In addition, fentanyl, a synthetic opioid unrelated to morphine, has also been shown to inhibit natural killer cell function during the perioperative period.[14] There are even data that suggest that morphine may play a proangiogenic role and promote breast tumor growth.[15] Given the role that cellular immunity plays in regulating cancer cell growth and spread, these data create concern for those treating patients with cancer with morphine, with fentanyl, and by extension other opioid medications.[16] However, the interplay of surgery, acute pain, and opioid medications on the stress response and subsequent immunomodulation is complex and not yet completely understood.[17]

Not all studies are in agreement with the effects of opioids on immune function and cancer proliferation. One study in direct contrast measured natural killer cell activity in humans after fentanyl administration and found that natural killer cytotoxicity rapidly increased following exposure to fentanyl.[18] Another study, this time in rats, found that morphine administration seemed to block metastasis following surgery but not in the animals without surgery.[19] These data seem to indicate that opioid medications themselves can help mitigate some of the immune effects of surgery, particularly if the opioids are used to treat pain, which itself may be immunossuppressive.[17]

REGIONAL ANESTHESIA AND LOCAL ANESTHETIC EFFECTS ON IMMUNOSUPPRESSION

Regional anesthesia has long been considered an alternative to general anesthesia (GA) or a supplement with particular use in the postoperative period. Although opioids have a complex interaction with the stress response following surgery and the subsequent immune effects, regional anesthesia when using a local anesthetic-based solution has been shown repeatedly to attenuate the surgical stress response.[20] Furthermore, both intraoperative and postoperative use of a thoracic epidural for abdominal surgery has been shown to reduce the stress-induced immunosuppression even more than postoperative epidural use alone.[21] As regional anesthesia is able to block the neuroendocrine stress response and subsequent decrease in cellular immunity, it follows that regional anesthesia may reduce cancer cell metastasis in the perioperative period; this has been shown in a rat model with spinal anesthesia decreasing the rate of metastasis by 70% following surgery.[22] In addition, the perioperative use of regional anesthesia-analgesia may result in decreased use of other agents (eg, inhalational agents, opioids) that may promote conditions more favorable to tumor growth.

Although regional anesthesia with use of local anesthetics can decrease the surgical stress response, local anesthetic agents themselves can affect tumor cell growth. Lidocaine, at least in vitro, appears to have an inhibitory effect on the epidermal growth factor receptor.[23] This inhibitory effect has been shown to reduce the growth of a human tongue cancer cell line.[24] Ropivacaine, in addition to lidocaine, has also been shown to have some antitumor activity as well.[25] Although this research is promising, more data are necessary to further elucidate any potential benefits of local anesthetics in human cancer treatment.

STUDIES INVESTIGATING THE RELATIONSHIP BETWEEN REGIONAL ANESTHESIA AND CANCER RECURRENCE

There are several studies that have examined the relationship between regional anesthesia-analgesia and cancer recurrence (**Table 1**). All of these studies have been published within the past decade and in essence are observational studies (ie, prospective/retrospective cohort from a database or a reanalysis of data from previously published randomized controlled studies). There is no definitive answer to this question because there are significant methodologic flaws in the available studies,

Table 1
Summary data of available studies examining cancer recurrence and regional anesthesia

Study, Year	Type of Study	Population (RA/GA)	Surgery	Hazard Ratio	95% CI	Result
Exadaktylos et al,[26] 2006	OBS	129 (50/79)	Breast	0.21	0.06–0.71	+
Biki et al,[27] 2008	OBS	225 (123/102)	Prostate	0.43	0.22–0.83	+
Christopherson-I et al,[28] 2008	RCT	177 (85/92)	Colorectal (for nonmetastatic CA)	0.216	0.065–0.718	+
Christopherson-II et al,[28] 2008	RCT	177 (85/92)	Colorectal (for metastatic CA)	0.699	0.395–1.236	–
Gottschalk et al,[40] 2010	RCT	509 (256/253)	Colorectal	0.82	0.49–1.35	±
Ismail et al,[32] 2010	OBS	132 (63/69)	Cervical	0.95	0.54–1.67	–
Tsui et al,[31] 2010	RCT	99 (49/50)	Prostate	1.33	0.64–2.77	–
Wuethrich et al,[41] 2010	OBS	261 (103/158)	Prostate	0.45	0.27–0.75	±
de Oliveira et al,[29] 2011	OBS	182 (55/127)	GYN	0.37	0.19–0.73	±
Gupta-I et al,[33] 2011	OBS	453 (360/93)	Colorectal (colon CA)	0.82	0.30–2.19	–
Gupta-II et al,[33] 2011	OBS	388 (295/93)	Colorectal (rectal CA)	0.45	0.22–0.90	+
Myles et al,[34] 2011	RCT	503 (230/216)	Intra-abdominal	0.95	0.76–1.17	–
Day et al,[39] 2012	RCT	424 (251/173)	Colorectal	n/a	n/a	–
Lai et al,[35] 2012	OBS	179 (62/117)	Hepatic	3.66	2.59–5.15	–
Binczak et al,[38] 2013	RCT	132 (69/63)	Intra-abdominal	1.3	0.8–2.0	–
Lacassie et al,[37] 2013	OBS	80 (37/43)	Ovarian	0.74	0.36–1.49	–
Merquiol et al,[30] 2013	OBS	271 (160/111)	Head & neck	0.49	0.25–0.96	+
Wuethrich et al,[36] 2013	OBS	148 (67/81)	Prostate	1.17	0.63–2.17	–

+: suggests regional anesthesia (RA) decreases cancer recurrence compared with GA.
–: suggests RA has does not decrease cancer recurrence versus GA.
Abbreviations: CA, cancer; CI, confidence interval; GYN, gynecologic; N/A, not available; OBS, observational study.
Data from Refs.[26–41]

although there are several ongoing randomized controlled trials (RCTs) that ultimately may provide more robust data on this topic.

Regional Anesthesia Does Improve Cancer Recurrence

The association between perioperative regional anesthesia-analgesia and cancer recurrence has been demonstrated in a handful of clinical studies. Exadaktylos and colleagues[26] in 2006 were the first to suggest that regional anesthesia-analgesia may help reduce the risk of cancer recurrence. This study was retrospective and evaluated the medical records of 129 patients undergoing surgical treatment of breast cancer with mastectomy and axillary clearance. Patients with paravertebral anesthesia and analgesia combined with GA were compared with those with GA and postoperative morphine analgesia, with regards to recurrence-free and metastasis-free survival for up to a 37-month follow-up period. The regional anesthesia-analgesia group had a higher long-term survival rate: 94% survival at both 24 and 36 months versus 82% and 77%, respectively, for the morphine analgesia group.

Biki and colleagues[27] in 2008 published another retrospective review investigating prostate cancer recurrence in patients undergoing open radical prostatectomy with either GA with epidural anesthesia-analgesia or GA with postoperative opioid analgesia. Similarly, this group found that the regional anesthesia-analgesia group had an estimated 57% lower risk of biochemical cancer recurrence. Long-term postoperative survival after colon cancer resection using GA with or without epidural anesthesia-analgesia was also studied by Christopherson and colleagues.[28] This study was a reanalysis of a previous RCT that looked at short-term mortality and morbidity between the 2 treatments; patients with and without metastases were evaluated separately. In this study, epidural anesthesia did enhance survival, but only for those without metastases before 1.46 years. For those with metastases, epidural supplementation did not affect survival.

de Oliveira and colleagues[29] looked more closely at the timing of epidural anesthesia-analgesia usage and its effect on ovarian cancer recurrence. Time to recurrence was compared between groups who received epidural anesthesia-analgesia intraoperatively and postoperatively, postoperatively alone, or not at all. The mean time to recurrence for the intraoperative regional anesthesia-analgesia group was longer at 73 months, compared with the 33-month and 38-month means of the epidural postoperative group or no-epidural group, respectively.

More recently, in 2013, Merquiol and colleagues[30] retrospectively looked at cervical epidural anesthesia with head and neck cancer recurrence. Sixty-five matched pairs who underwent larynx or hypopharynx cancer surgery were examined. Those with combined GA and cervical epidural anesthesia had a 68% 5-year cancer-free survival, compared with 37% for the GA-alone group. This study again suggests that regional anesthesia-analgesia, by blunting the stress response and by preserving the immune response during the time of surgery, has long-term effects on cancer recurrence.

Regional Anesthesia Does Not Improve Cancer Recurrence

Although initially there were many studies that showed a positive association with regional anesthesia-analgesia and tumor recurrence, more recent studies have not been as favorable. Several studies based on reanalyzed data from RCTs as well as observational studies have found there to be no difference in cancer recurrence with or without the use of regional anesthesia-analgesia.

Tsui and colleagues[31] undertook a reanalysis of an RCT of patients who underwent radical prostatectomy under GA with and without epidural anesthesia. Prostate cancer recurrence was then determined after a long-term follow-up chart review between the

2 groups. With a hazard ratio of 1.33 for the study group compared with the control group, they found no significant difference in disease-free survival at median follow-up of 4.5 years.

In a retrospective cohort study, Ismail and colleagues[32] looked to see if the use of neuraxial anesthesia during the first session of brachytherapy would affect the progression of cervical cancer. Compared with the use of GA, neuraxial anesthesia did not reduce the risk of local or systemic recurrence. In addition, long-term mortality from tumor recurrence and all-cause mortality were not affected by the type of anesthetic chosen for the procedure.

Gupta and colleagues[33] retrospectively reviewed 655 patients having colorectal cancer surgery with either epidural analgesia or intravenous patient-controlled analgesia. Interestingly, the epidural analgesia group had decreased all-cause mortality after rectal, but not colon, cancer surgery. Age greater than 72, patient-controlled analgesia rather than epidural usage, and cancer stages 2 and 3 had a higher risk for death after rectal cancer surgery. The colon cancer group showed no difference between the 2 groups of analgesia.

A reanalysis was done on data collected for 503 patients who underwent major abdominal surgery for cancer using GA with or without epidural blockade for a minimum 3 postoperative days.[34] In this study, Myles and colleagues found the median time to recurrence or death was 2.8 years and 2.6 years for the control and epidural groups, respectively. They concluded that epidural anesthesia-analgesia was not associated with a decrease in cancer recurrence.

Lai and colleagues[35] actually found a negative association with epidural anesthesia used for patients undergoing percutaneous radiofrequency ablation for small hepatocellular carcinoma. This retrospective analysis found a statistically significant lower cancer-free survival in the epidural anesthesia group compared with the GA group. However, overall mortality between the 2 groups was not different.

Another retrospective study evaluated 148 patients who underwent retropubic radical prostatectomy with either GA and intraoperative/postoperative epidural analgesia or GA with ketorolac-morphine analgesia.[36] With a median observation time of 14 years, Wuethrich and colleagues[36] found no difference in biochemical recurrence, local and distant recurrence-free, cancer-specific survival, and overall survival between the 2 groups.

Lacassie and colleagues[37] found similar results for patients who received epidural anesthesia-analgesia with GA for advanced ovarian cancer removal. They analyzed data from 11 years of surgeries, using propensity scoring methods, matching, and inverse weighting to compare time to recurrence and overall survival. No benefit was seen with the use of epidural anesthesia-analgesia in this patient population.

In a reanalysis of data comparing epidural anesthesia-analgesia to fentanyl followed by continuous subcutaneous morphine for major intra-abdominal surgery for cancer removal, Binczak and colleagues[38] also investigated the influence of regional analgesia on recurrence-free and overall survival. Although they found a general trend in favor of the epidural group, these results did not reach statistical significance over the 17-year median follow-up.

Day and colleagues[39] retrospectively looked at patients undergoing laparoscopic colorectal resection for adenocarcinoma with either epidural, spinal, or morphine patient-controlled analgesia for their primary postoperative analgesia. Interestingly, the epidural group had a longer median length of stay. There was also no difference in overall survival or disease-free survival at 5 years between the 3 groups.

Regional Anesthesia May or May Not Improve Cancer Recurrence

Some studies have had mixed results wherein subpopulations are found to have a positive association between perioperative regional anesthesia-analgesia and cancer recurrence. In 2010, Gottschalk and colleagues[40] looked at the records of 506 patients who underwent colorectal cancer surgery, either with or without perioperative epidural analgesia. Although there was no overall association between epidural analgesia use and cancer recurrence in the initial analysis, a post-hoc analysis did reveal that there may be some benefit for patients older than 64 years.

In a nonrandomized, retrospective review of 261 patients, Wuethrich and colleagues[41] studied the effect of GA with or without intraoperative/postoperative epidural anesthesia-analgesia for retropubic radical prostatectomy. No difference was found for biochemical recurrence-free survival, cancer-specific survival, or overall survival between the 2 anesthetic choices. However, clinical progress-free survival was improved for the epidural analgesia group.

META-ANALYSES

There have been limited attempts to perform a meta-analysis based on the available studies and literature. However, the lack of data as well as type of studies done, which are mainly observational and secondary analyses of RCTs, makes it difficult to draw definite associations. This challenge is compounded by the heterogeneity of data, such as the numerous types of surgeries and tumors included, as well as the many definitions of "recurrence."

In 2012, Chen and colleagues[42] performed a meta-analysis of studies that looked at the effect of regional anesthesia-analgesia on both overall survival and recurrence-free survival. They found 14 total studies, which contained 18 substudies. Seven of these focused on overall survival analysis and 11 focused on recurrence-free survival. For overall survival, their analysis favored epidural anesthesia compared with GA alone, especially in colorectal cancer surgery. With regards to recurrence-free survival, there was no statistically significant association with epidural anesthesia. The results suggest that although epidural anesthesia-analgesia was associated with improved overall survival, it did not contribute to cancer control.

Cata and colleagues[43] in 2013 performed a systematic review on the use of regional anesthesia and postoperative analgesia to improve cancer-related survival after surgery. Thirteen articles fit their inclusion criteria, all of which were retrospective in nature. Because of the high heterogeneity of the studies and the lack of RCTs, the authors thought that a meta-analysis would not be appropriate. The authors found mixed results for gastrointestinal and genitourinary surgery and only one relevant positive study on regional breast cancer. The conclusion was that despite basic science suggestions that regional anesthesia may reduce cancer recurrence, there was a paucity of actual clinical evidence in support of this theory.

SURGICAL SITE INFECTIONS AND REGIONAL ANESTHESIA

SSIs continue to be one of the most serious complications during the perioperative period. Roughly 157,500 SSIs occur annually, resulting in increased length of stay and hospital readmission.[44] Overall incidence of SSI is thought to be around 1% to 3%, but the risk for colorectal surgery can be as high as 15% to 35%.[45] Although many SSIs can be prevented, patients that do develop a SSI have a significantly increased mortality compared with patients who do not develop a SSI.[46]

The immunologic principles affecting perioperative immunosuppression and cancer recurrence are also applicable to that for SSI. A common approach for preventing SSIs involves maintaining the immune system and improving tissue oxygenation, which helps maintain neutrophil function. As such, several interventions have been shown to decrease SSIs, including maintaining normothermia and limiting blood transfusions.[47] Regional anesthesia has also been suggested as a possible means to limit SSIs. As mentioned previously, surgery stimulates the stress response, which can result in immunosuppression in the perioperative period. Uncontrolled pain can trigger the sympathetic nervous system, resulting in vasoconstriction as well. By mitigating the stress response, regional anesthesia may be another potential method to help reduce SSIs.

Several studies have looked directly at the relationship between regional anesthesia and SSIs. In 2010, Chang and colleagues[48] published a retrospective study comparing SSI rates over a 30-day period in patients undergoing either primary total hip or knee replacements. They demonstrated that GA patients had a slightly more than 2 times higher rate of SSIs than those receiving an epidural or spinal anesthetic. A separate retrospective study, this time in an obstetric population undergoing caesarean delivery, again favored neuraxial anesthesia with regards to reduced SSIs in a 30-day period.[49] The GA population tended to be older as well as more often diabetic, preeclamptic, and having signs of fetal distress. When adjusted for these patient characteristics and others, GA still had a 2.21 significantly higher odds of SSI. Both of the above studies, although favoring regional anesthesia over GA in terms of SSI rates, are limited by their retrospective nature. The practitioners' reasons for selection of GA over regional anesthesia are unknown and could have affected the results.

An additional retrospective study published in 2011 sought to examine if there was a morbidity and mortality benefit from postoperative epidural analgesia in 1470 patients.[50] In this study, however, patients with epidurals did not benefit in terms of a difference in SSIs. Another earlier study, this time a systematic review examining postoperative morbidity and mortality with epidural or spinal anesthesia, also found no difference in SSI when compared with GA.[51]

SUMMARY

Perioperative immune function is important for the prevention of cancer recurrence and SSI in surgical patients who typically experience a transient period of immunosuppression. Although there are many potential inputs into perioperative immunosuppression, the use of regional anesthesia-analgesia with a local anesthetic-based regimen may attenuate the surgical stress response and preserve perioperative immune function. Other advantages of using perioperative regional anesthesia-analgesia are the decrease in the use of opioids and inhalation agents, which may contribute to perioperative immunosuppression. Despite the theoretic benefits of regional anesthesia-analgesia in decreasing cancer recurrence and SSIs, currently available data are equivocal.

REFERENCES

1. Dunn GP, Old LJ, Schreiber RD. The immunobiology of cancer immunosurveillance and immunoediting. Immunity 2004;21(2):137–48.
2. Grulich AE, van Leeuwen MT, Falster MO, et al. Incidence of cancers in people with HIV/AIDS compared with immunosuppressed transplant recipients: a meta-analysis. Lancet 2007;370(9581):59–67.

3. Vajdic CM, van Leeuwen MT. Cancer incidence and risk factors after solid organ transplantation. Int J Cancer 2009;125(8):1747–54.
4. Engels EA, Pfeiffer RM, Fraumeni JF Jr, et al. Spectrum of cancer risk among US solid organs transplants recipients. JAMA 2011;306(17):1891–901.
5. Imai K, Matsuyama S, Miyake S, et al. Natural cytotoxic activity of peripheral-blood lymphocytes and cancer incidence: an 11-year follow-up study of a general population. Lancet 2000;356(9244):1795–9.
6. Ben-Eliyahu S. The promotion of tumor metastasis by surgery and stress: immunological basis and implications for psychoneuroimmunology. Brain Behav Immun 2003;17(Suppl 1):S27–36.
7. Page GG. Surgery-induced immunosuppression and postoperative pain management. AACN Clin Issues 2005;16(3):302–9.
8. Koda K, Saito N, Takiguchi N, et al. Preoperative natural killer cell activity: correlation with distant metastases in curatively research colorectal carcinomas. Int Surg 1997;82(2):190–3.
9. Takeuchi H, Maehara Y, Tokunaga E, et al. Prognostic significance of natural killer cell activity in patients with gastric carcinoma: a multivariate analysis. Am J Gastroenterol 2001;96(2):574–8.
10. Tsuchiya Y, Sawada S, Yoshioka I, et al. Increased surgical stress promotes tumor metastasis. Surgery 2003;133(5):547–55.
11. Lacy AM, Garcia-Valdecasas JC, Delgado S, et al. Laparoscopy-assisted colectomy versus open colectomy for treatment of non-metastatic colon cancer: a randomised trial. Lancet 2002;359:2224–9.
12. Page GG, Blakely WP, Ben-Eliyahu S. Evidence that postoperative pain is a mediator for the tumor-promoting effects of surgery in rats. Pain 2001;90(1–2):191–9.
13. Yeager MP, Colacchio TA, Yu CT, et al. Morphine inhibits spontaneous and cytokine-enhanced natural killer cell cytotoxicity in volunteers. Anesthesiology 1995;83(3):500–8.
14. Beilin B, Shavit Y, Hart J, et al. Effects of anesthesia based on large versus small doses of fentanyl on natural killer cell cytotoxicity in the perioperative period. Anesth Analg 1996;82(3):492–7.
15. Gupta K, Kshirsagar S, Chang L, et al. Morphine stimulates angiogenesis by activating proangiogenic and survival-promoting signaling and promotes breast tumor growth. Cancer Res 2002;62(15):4491–8.
16. Afsharimani B, Cabot PJ, Parat MO. Morphine use in cancer surgery. Front Pharmacol 2011;2:46.
17. Page GG. Immunologic effects of opioids in the presence or absence of pain. J Pain Symptom Manage 2005;29:S25–31.
18. Yeager MP, Procopio MA, DeLeo JA, et al. Intravenous fentanyl increases natural killer cell cytotoxicity and circulating CD16(+) lymphocytes in humans. Anesth Analg 2002;94(1):94–9.
19. Page GG, Ben-Eliyahu S, Yirmiya R, et al. Morphine attenuates surgery-induced enhancement of metastatic colonization in rats. Pain 1993;54(1):21–8.
20. Liu S, Carpenter RL, Neal JM. Epidural anesthesia and analgesia: their role in postoperative outcome. Anesthesiology 1995;82(6):1474–506.
21. Ahlers O, Nachtigall I, Lenze J, et al. Intraoperative thoracic epidural anaesthesia attenuates stress-induced immunosuppression in patients undergoing major abdominal surgery. Br J Anaesth 2008;101(6):781–7.
22. Bar-Yosef S, Melamed R, Page GG, et al. Attenuation of the tumor-promoting effect of surgery by spinal blockade in rats. Anesthesiology 2001;94(6):1066–73.

23. Mammoto T, Higashiyama S, Mukai M, et al. Infiltration anesthetic lidocaine inhibits cancer cell invasion by modulating ectodomain shedding of heparin-binding epidermal growth factor-like growth factor (HB-EGF). J Cell Physiol 2002;192(3):351–8.

24. Sakaguchi M, Kuroda Y, Hirose M. The antiproliferative effect of lidocaine on human tongue cancer cells with inhibition of the activity of epidermal growth factor receptor. Anesth Analg 2006;102(4):1103–7.

25. Santamaria LB, Schifilliti D, La Torre D, et al. Drugs of anaesthesia and cancer. Surg Oncol 2010;19(2):63–81.

26. Exadaktylos AK, Buggy DJ, Moriarty DC, et al. Can anesthetic technique for primary breast cancer surgery affect recurrence or metastasis? Anesthesiology 2006;105(4):660–4.

27. Biki B, Mascha E, Moriarty DC, et al. Anesthetic technique for radical prostatectomy surgery affects cancer recurrence: a retrospective analysis. Anesthesiology 2008;109(2):180–7.

28. Christopherson R, James KE, Tableman M, et al. Long-term survival after colon cancer surgery: a variation associated with choice of anesthesia. Anesth Analg 2008;107(1):325–32.

29. de Oliveira GS Jr, Ahmad S, Schink JC, et al. Intraoperative neuraxial anesthesia but not postoperative neuraxial analgesia is associated with increased relapse-free survival in ovarian cancer patients after primary cytoreductive surgery. Reg Anesth Pain Med 2011;36(3):271–7.

30. Merquiol F, Montelimard AS, Nourissat A, et al. Cervical epidural anesthesia is associated with increased cancer-free survival in laryngeal and hypopharyngeal cancer surgery: a retrospective propensity-matched analysis. Reg Anesth Pain Med 2013;38(5):398–402.

31. Tsui BC, Rashiq S, Schopflocher D, et al. Epidural anesthesia and cancer recurrence rates after radical prostatectomy. Can J Anaesth 2010;57(2):107–12.

32. Ismail H, Ho KM, Narayan K, et al. Effect of neuraxial anaesthesia on tumour progression in cervical cancer patients treated with brachytherapy: a retrospective cohort study. Br J Anaesth 2010;105(2):145–9.

33. Gupta A, Björnsson A, Fredriksson M, et al. Reduction in mortality after epidural anaesthesia and analgesia in patients undergoing rectal but not colonic cancer surgery: a retrospective analysis of data from 655 patients in central Sweden. Br J Anaesth 2011;107(2):164–70.

34. Myles PS, Peyton P, Silbert B, et al. Perioperative epidural analgesia for major abdominal surgery for cancer and recurrence-free survival: randomised trial. BMJ 2011;342:d1491.

35. Lai R, Peng Z, Chen D, et al. The effects of anesthetic technique on cancer recurrence in percutaneous radiofrequency ablation of small hepatocellular carcinoma. Anesth Analg 2012;114(2):290–6.

36. Wuethrich PY, Thalmann GN, Studer UE, et al. Epidural analgesia during open radical prostatectomy does not improve long-term cancer-related outcome: a retrospective study in patients with advanced prostate cancer. PLoS One 2013;8(8):e72873.

37. Lacassie HJ, Cartagena J, Branes J, et al. The relationship between neuraxial anesthesia and advanced ovarian cancer-related outcomes in the Chilean population. Anesth Analg 2013;117(3):653–60.

38. Binczak M, Tournay E, Billard V, et al. Major abdominal surgery for cancer: does epidural analgesia have a long-term effect on recurrence-free and overall survival? Ann Fr Anesth Reanim 2013;32(5):e81–8.

39. Day A, Smith R, Jourdan I, et al. Retrospective analysis of the effect of postoperative analgesia on survival in patients after laparoscopic resection of colorectal cancer. Br J Anaesth 2012;109(2):185–90.
40. Gottschalk A, Ford JG, Regelin CC, et al. Association between epidural analgesia and cancer recurrence after colorectal cancer surgery. Anesthesiology 2010;113(1):27–34.
41. Wuethrich PY, Hsu Schmitz SF, Kessler TM, et al. Potential influence of the anesthetic technique used during open radical prostatectomy on prostate cancer-related outcome: a retrospective study. Anesthesiology 2010;113(3):570–6.
42. Chen WK, Miao CH. The effect of anesthetic technique on survival in human cancers: a meta-analysis of retrospective and prospective studies. PLoS One 2013;8(2):e56540.
43. Cata JP, Hernandez M, Lewis VO, et al. Can regional anesthesia and analgesia prolong cancer survival after orthopaedic oncologic surgery? Clin Orthop Relat Res 2014;472:1434–41.
44. Scott RD. U.S. Centers for Disease Control and Prevention. 2009. Available at: www.cdc.gov/HAI/surveillance/index.html. Accessed September 16, 2014.
45. Gervaz P, Bandiera-Clerc C, Buchs NC, et al. Scoring system to predict the risk of surgical-site infection after colorectal resection. Br J Surg 2012;99:589–95.
46. Anderson DJ, Kaye KS, Classon D, et al. Strategies to prevent surgical site infections in acute care hospitals. Infect Control Hosp Epidemiol 2008;29(Suppl 1):S51–61.
47. Kavanagh T, Buggy D. Can anaesthetic technique effect postoperative outcome? Curr Opin Anesthesiol 2012;25(2):185–98.
48. Chang CC, Lin HC, Lin HW, et al. Anesthetic management and surgical site infection in total hip or knee replacement: a population based study. Anesthesiology 2010;113(2):279–84.
49. Tsai PS, Hsu CS, Fan YC, et al. General anaesthesia is associated with increased risk of surgical site infection after Caesarean delivery compared with neuraxial anaesthesia: a population based study. Br J Anaesth 2011;107(5):757–61.
50. Warschkow R, Steffen T, Luthi A, et al. Epidural analgesia in open resection of colorectal cancer: is there a clinical benefit? A retrospective study on 1470 patients. J Gastrointest Surg 2011;15(8):1386–93.
51. Rodgers A, Walker N, Schug S, et al. Reduction of postoperative mortality and morbidity with epidural or spinal anaesthesia: results from overview of randomized trials. BMJ 2000;321(7275):1493.

Developing a Multidisciplinary Fall Reduction Program for Lower-Extremity Joint Arthroplasty Patients

T. Edward Kim, MD[a,b],
Edward R. Mariano, MD, MAS (Clinical Research)[a,b],*

KEYWORDS

- Fall prevention • Fall reduction • Patient safety • Total joint replacement
- Regional anesthesia

KEY POINTS

- Total joint arthroplasty patients are at increased risk for postoperative falls, and anesthesiologists can provide leadership in promoting patient safety during the perioperative period.
- A multidisciplinary team approach is associated with greater success in implementing interventions and reducing fall rates.
- Multicomponent interventions that address risk factors specific to each hospital's total joint arthroplasty patients are essential to a successful fall reduction program.
- Making fall reduction interventions an integral and routine part of patient care is necessary for long-term changes.

Financial Support: None.
Conflict of Interest: Dr E.R. Mariano has received unrestricted funding paid to his institution for educational programs from I-Flow/Kimberly-Clark (Lake Forest, CA) and B Braun (Bethlehem, PA). These companies had absolutely no input into any aspect of the present study conceptualization, design, and implementation; data collection, analysis and interpretation; or manuscript preparation.
[a] Anesthesiology and Perioperative Care Service, VA Palo Alto Health Care System, 3801 Miranda Avenue (112A), Palo Alto, CA 94304, USA; [b] Department of Anesthesiology, Perioperative and Pain Medicine, Stanford University School of Medicine, 300 Pasteur Drive #H3580, Stanford, CA 94305, USA
* Corresponding author. Anesthesiology and Perioperative Care Service, VA Palo Alto Health Care System, 3801 Miranda Avenue (112A), Palo Alto, CA 94304.
E-mail address: emariano@stanford.edu

Anesthesiology Clin 32 (2014) 853–864
http://dx.doi.org/10.1016/j.anclin.2014.08.005
1932-2275/14/$ – see front matter Published by Elsevier Inc.

INTRODUCTION

Falls continue to occur frequently in the community, long-term care facilities, and hospitals, often leading to adverse events. In 2011, emergency departments in the United States treated 2.4 million adults with fall-related injuries, leading to 689,000 patient hospitalizations.[1] During a 2-year span in Australia, one in every six patients 70 years of age or older presented to the emergency department because of a fall, which averaged 4.4 falls per day, with 40% of subsequent hospitalizations caused by fractures.[2] The incidence of falls among hospitalized patients 65 years of age or older is close to three times the rate observed in the community.[3] For acute-care hospitals, fall rates (equal to total number of falls/number of occupied bed days × 1000) can range from 1.3 to 8.9 falls per 1000 hospital days, with higher rates in certain wards specializing in neurology, geriatrics, and physical rehabilitation.[4]

The Joint Commission (TJC) includes fall prevention as one of the national patient safety goals and requires each health care facility to effectuate a fall reduction program.[5] The increasing focus on inpatient fall reduction is justified. Falls can lead to physical injuries, anxiety and fear of future falls, and prolonged hospital stays.[4,6–9] In addition, the financial burden of falls on the health care system is not insignificant. In 2000, direct medical costs in the United States for nonfatal fall injuries were $19 billion.[10] The Centers for Medicare and Medicaid Services categorize inpatient falls as a hospital-acquired condition, leaving hospitals to shoulder the burden of costs associated with subsequent care.[11]

When considering lower-extremity total joint replacement surgeries, patients may incur additional risks compared with their nonsurgical counterparts because of potential gait and balance disturbances, effects of postoperative polypharmacy, intravascular volume status changes, and unfamiliarity with the hospital environment. This target patient population is of particular interest to anesthesiologists because 3.48 million total knee replacement procedures are estimated to be performed each year by 2030 in the United States.[12] Although the care of surgical patients by anesthesiologists has been defined traditionally in the preoperative and intraoperative periods, the increasing implementation of regional anesthesia techniques for acute pain medicine and the expanding perioperative role (perioperative surgical home concept)[13] are involving anesthesiologists more frequently in the management of postoperative outcomes and complications. Anesthesiologists are in a position to provide leadership in preventing falls and to collaborate with other health care providers to improve patient safety among total joint arthroplasty patients.

CURRENT GUIDELINES

Although falls are widespread in acute-care and long-term settings and recognized as a potential comorbidity, there has yet to be established a generally accepted or standardized fall reduction program for hospitals. Numerous studies have investigated the effectiveness of interventions or strategies singly or in combination[4,14]; however, the dynamic etiologies of, and variable circumstances surrounding, falls have precluded a program that can be universally applied to all patient care settings. In a 2001 fall prevention guideline published jointly by the American Geriatrics Society, British Geriatric Society, and American Academy of Orthopedic Surgeons, recommendations were provided mostly for community-dwellers and long-term care centers, but the panel concluded that further studies were necessary to outline fall prevention elements for acute-care hospitalized patients.[3] TJC outlines key elements that should be included in a fall reduction program (**Box 1**). Even though there is no defined program for total joint arthroplasty patients, previous investigations have addressed inpatient falls in

association between peripheral nerve blocks and inpatient falls.[25] In addition, patients who had neuraxial anesthesia as the primary intraoperative anesthetic were less likely to fall than patients who had general anesthesia alone.[25] Given the conflicting data regarding the potential association between regional anesthesia techniques and falls, further studies are needed especially in light of recent investigations that have identified functional benefits of certain peripheral nerve blocks. For example, the adductor canal block is a more selective peripheral nerve block of the lower extremity that targets the saphenous nerve and has been used for TKA postoperative pain management.[26] TKA patients with adductor canal blocks can ambulate greater distances[26] without equivalent muscle weakness when compared to patients with femoral nerve blocks.[27]

STRATEGIES AND INTERVENTIONS

For total joint arthroplasty patients in the acute postoperative period, preventing falls and/or injuries without interfering with physical and occupational rehabilitation is the highest safety priority. The selection of a tailored fall reduction program should be based on modifying risk factors identified for the local patient population. Previous investigations provide a general framework and examples of programs implemented in other hospitals. In a prospective study performed in an orthopedic ward, interventions that focused primarily on providing routine assistance to and from the restroom or commode led to a 40% decrease in overall fall rate and 65% reduction in fall-related injuries.[28] Before selecting the interventions, previous falls that occurred in the orthopedic ward were evaluated, and toileting activities were identified as one of the highest risk for falls. Subsequently, three of four interventions were aimed at increasing the awareness of and providing assistance with patient toileting needs. In another prospective cohort study, a multidisciplinary fall prevention program in an orthopedic hospital resulted in a 30% relative risk reduction in falls.[15] There were 11 patient interventions that were selected in a tiered system consisting of universal interventions for all patients and specific interventions reserved for high-risk patients. Although the selected interventions were different from the aforementioned study, the latter study also resulted in a decreased fall rate. Based on these two disparate but successful programs among postsurgical orthopedic patients, it can be concluded that interventions that address targeted risk factors are essential in designing a standardized fall reduction program.

In a clinical pathway that includes lower-extremity peripheral nerve blocks, especially perineural infusions during periods of ambulation, muscle weakness and knee instability should be addressed. Potential options include reducing local anesthetic total dose[29,30] and/or pausing infusions before physical or occupational therapy and using mechanical devices. For example, in a retrospective study at a single institution, fall rate was reduced after implementation of knee immobilizer braces in TKA patients with continuous femoral perineural infusions.[31]

It is outside the scope of this article to review every potential intervention for fall reduction. Current systematic reviews and meta-analyses provide descriptions of fall prevention strategies and have identified interventions that are commonly included in fall prevention programs. Frequently applied interventions include fall risk assessment, education for patients and staff, bed-alarms, appropriate footwear, bedside visual aids, toileting schedules, medication review, postfall evaluations, and risk alert system.[4,6,16,32] Although certain interventions have been studied individually, research suggests that fall reduction programs with multifactorial components are more successful in decreasing fall rates than a single intervention.[4,8,33]

IMPLEMENTATION

After individual components of a fall reduction program are identified, the success of the program depends largely on how it is introduced into clinical practice. The impact of the interventions on staff work duties should be assessed. Education and training of care providers regarding their roles and responsibilities are critical before introducing the program.[15,28] Furthermore, a trial period to pilot interventions can provide valuable information about the program's feasibility and effectiveness.[34] Clearly delineating responsibilities, ensuring availability and accessibility of resources and tools, and receiving feedback from bedside providers can promote implementation of the program and facilitate the incorporation of new interventions into pre-existing clinical practices. The commitment to patient safety and fall prevention may be the fundamental element that leads to the success of the interventions.[35]

SUSTAINABILITY

Part of the fall reduction program should include strategies that encourage and support daily application of the implemented interventions. Continued adherence to the program is necessary to effectuate long-term changes[32] and is integral to promoting a culture of safety.[35] Much like the selection of individual interventions, there can be variability in adherence strategies. The ultimate goal, however, is to integrate the program into routine patient care rather than a temporary or special project. Although there are insufficient data to recommend the most effective methods to ensure a program's sustainability, the systematic review by Hempel and colleagues[32] highlights the following strategies: "audit and feedback on adherence to processes of care, monitoring and disseminating fall data, and integrating risk assessments into an electronic health record." Another systematic review also found that fall reduction programs often include reviews after falls.[6] At the authors' hospital, a postfall huddle is performed shortly after a fall to evaluate the patient's risk factors and circumstances surrounding the incident. A thorough review may lead to specific modifications for that patient or more global changes to the fall reduction program. Fall champions are also assigned to assist with ongoing efforts. For each shift, a fall champion who is familiar with the interventions is a valuable resource to encourage and evaluate the application of the fall reduction program and can help identify challenges. The fall champion can enhance communication between bedside providers and the fall team, assist in training newly hired staff, ensure timely postfall documentation, and participate in fall rounds. The hospital-wide fall prevention team meets every month to review fall risks and etiologies, implemented interventions, and fall-related policies. Fall data are reported monthly and are accessible through a hospital database. Regular assessment of fall rates among total joint arthroplasty patients is a barometer of the program's success and can validate continued efforts.

AN EXAMPLE OF SELECTING INTERVENTIONS FOR A FALL REDUCTION PROGRAM

At the authors' hospital, total joint arthroplasty patients are admitted postoperatively to an open surgical or rehabilitation unit and not an exclusive orthopedic unit. Subsequently, when the fall reduction program was being developed, universal fall prevention strategies were applied to all admitted patients irrespective of diagnoses or surgery. The clinical pathway for joint replacement surgery at the time included a continuous femoral nerve or fascia iliaca catheter infusion for TKA or THA, respectively, as part of a multimodal analgesic protocol. Patients were expected to ambulate with PT/OT on postoperative day 1, and to minimize muscle weakness, peripheral nerve infusions were paused several hours before the first session of physical therapy.

The potential risk of peripheral nerve blocks and falls provided an opportunity for the regional anesthesia and acute pain service to be an integral part of reinforcing fall prevention efforts. After taking the steps shown in **Fig. 1** to identify desired components for a fall reduction program, the following interventions were selected: preoperative fall education for patients by a member of the regional anesthesia team, fall risk assessment by nurses using the Morse Fall Scale, fall risk alert by PT/OT after each session, bedside fall risk sign, and bed-exit alarms.

Education

For total joint arthroplasty patients, Mandl and colleagues[19] observed the need for improved patient education, particularly to inform patients about the risks associated with toileting activities. The implementation of a successful program in an orthopedic hospital by Galbraith and colleagues[15] included fall risk education for high-risk patients. Even as a single intervention, patient education may decrease fall rates. In a study performed in a hospital with acute and subacute wards, of which one was an orthopedic unit, the implementation of a multimedia education program taught by trained health care providers reduced the rate of falls.[36] For TKA patients, a preoperative one-on-one education program during the routine preoperative surgical clinic visit reduced the number of in-hospital falls[37]; although femoral nerve blocks with or without sciatic nerve blocks were part of the clinical pathway, no falls were observed in the study group despite a higher rate of sciatic nerve block use.

At the authors' hospital, fall education is provided to the patient and family members on the day of surgery before receiving a peripheral nerve block. The decision was

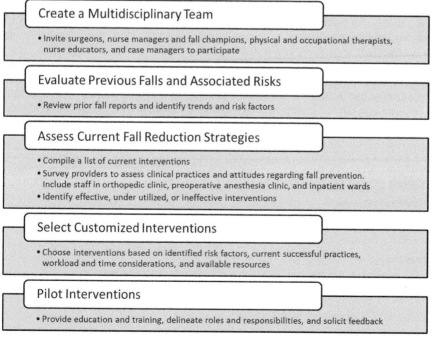

Fig. 1. Steps to selecting interventions for a fall reduction program.

made to conduct the education session on the day of surgery to ensure that patients were instructed by a member of the regional anesthesia and acute pain medicine team who manages the patient's postoperative pain. A standardized Fall Prevention Education Form is used for all patients, which includes an assessment of the patient's awareness of his or her fall risk after surgery, explanation of the anticipated effects of a peripheral nerve block, instructions on how patients can empower themselves from falling, and identification of interventions (ie, fall reduction program) that the hospital staff will implement during the hospitalization. The patient and a member of the regional anesthesiology and acute pain medicine team both sign the form to ensure understanding and promote adherence to the described protocol. This form is then posted in the patient's hospital room as a physical reminder and is reviewed daily during pain rounds.

Fall Risk Assessment Tools

A standardized assessment tool can identify a patient's potential risk factors, allow customization of interventions (eg, moving a patient to a room closer to nursing station to facilitate more frequent checks), and facilitate timely documentation and communication of risks to other health providers. There are many assessment tools available (**Box 2**). Common elements of assessment tools include identification of risk factors, such as history of falls; disturbances in ambulation, gait, strength, or balance; changes in mental status; toileting needs; comorbidities; and medications. Regardless of the assessment tool that is incorporated, proper implementation requires training and education of staff; in addition, guidelines regarding their use (eg, frequency of assessment) are encouraged. Although fall assessment tools are frequently used, it should be noted that identifying risk factors may not necessarily predict or prevent falls when they are used in a general patient population.[4,34] The potential time and resources required to implement an assessment tool in clinical practice should be considered.

At the authors' hospital, the Morse Fall Scale is used by nurses to assess TKA and THA patients' fall risks. The Morse Fall Scale is a commonly used assessment tool,[32] and was selected because of its generalized applicability and nurses' familiarity with the assessment as one of the pre-existing universal fall prevention strategies.

Alert System

Alert systems can include fall risk wristbands and signs in the patient's room and bathroom. Although fall risk identification bracelets were not shown to decrease fall rates as a single intervention,[38] systematic reviews indicate that an alert system is

---

Box 2
Examples of fall assessment tools used in published studies

ADAPT Fall Assessment

Berryman Predisposition for Falling

Hendrich II Fall Risk Model

Innes Score

Morse Fall Scale

Schmid Fall Risk Assessment

St. Thomas Risk Assessment Tool (STRATIFY)

Timed Up and Go Test

commonly included in multicomponent fall prevention programs and may contribute to decreasing the number of falls when used with other fall prevention strategies.[6,32] Signs can act as a reminder to patients, family members, and staff about the patient's risks and reinforce key fall prevention strategies that were discussed during the pre-operative education session. In the authors' hospital, the rooms occupied by total joint replacement patients have a large sign that states "Don't Fall, Call Your Nurse" in the shape and color of a STOP sign to remind patients to ask for assistance when they need to get out of bed, stand from a chair, ambulate, or use the bathroom. This sign is intentionally placed directly across the patient's line of sight, often underneath the television.

Another alert system used at our hospital is to designate the patient's permissible ambulation status on the patient's identification wristband using a color scheme. PT/OTs assess patients after each rehabilitation session and place one of three colored stickers on the wristband. A red sticker indicates that a patient is not to be out of bed. A yellow sticker signifies a patient can ambulate, but only with a nurse or PT/OT and an assistive device. A green sticker signals that a patient has been dis-charged by PT/OT and can ambulate using a recommended assistive device. The ad-vantages of a colored designation include easy identification of a patient's ambulation level and enhanced communication of a patient's status without having to contact PT/OT or look in the chart.

Bed-Exit Alarm

Similar to risk identification wristbands, bed-exit alarms as a single intervention have not shown to reduce fall rates[39,40] but may have a role in a multicomponent fall reduc-tion program, especially in acute-care hospitals with a multidisciplinary team.[41–43] Bed-exit alarms can remind patients to call for assistance and alert nurses when pa-tients are mobilizing or have fallen out of bed; however, false alarms and cost can be potential challenges. To ensure compliance with use, education and training should be provided before implementation.

Preliminary Results

As part of our review process, fall numbers were examined 1 year before and following the initiation of the fall reduction program. The combined fall rate for TKA and THA pa-tients in the surgical ward before and after the program was 4.4 falls versus 2.2 falls per 1000 hospital days. The preprogram period included the trial period. It should be noted that there was a change in the clinical practice for TKA patients 4 months before implementation of the fall reduction program. Femoral nerve catheters for TKA were replaced by adductor canal catheters,[26] and local anesthetic infusions were not paused postoperatively before physical or occupational therapy sessions. There were no changes in infusion rate or drug concentration. There were no changes in clinical practice for the total hip patients.

SUMMARY

With the anticipated increase in the number of total joint arthroplasty surgeries and associated fall risks, a fall reduction program can provide greater safety for patients in the postoperative period. Although further prospective studies are needed among total joint arthroplasty patients, there is sufficient evidence to show that a successful fall reduction program can be implemented. Common components to date include a multidisciplinary team, multicomponent interventions specific to the risks associated with TKA and THA patients, education of patients and staff, and strategies to promote adherence to the program.

REFERENCES

1. Centers for Disease Control and Prevention NCfIPaC. Web–based injury statistics query and reporting system (WISQARS). Available at: http://www.cdc.gov/HomeandRecreationalSafety/Falls/fallcost.html. Accessed March 12, 2014.
2. Close JC, Lord SR, Antonova EJ, et al. Older people presenting to the emergency department after a fall: a population with substantial recurrent healthcare use. Emerg Med J 2012;29:742–7.
3. Guideline for the prevention of falls in older persons. American Geriatrics Society, British Geriatrics Society, and American Academy of Orthopaedic Surgeons Panel on Falls Prevention. J Am Geriatr Soc 2001;49:664–72.
4. Oliver D, Healey F, Haines TP. Preventing falls and fall-related injuries in hospitals. Clin Geriatr Med 2010;26:645–92.
5. Commission TJ. National patient safety goals effective January 1, 2014: Home Care Accreditation Program. Available at: http://www.jointcommission.org/assets/1/6/OME_NPSG_Chapter_2014.pdf. Accessed March 12, 2014.
6. Miake-Lye IM, Hempel S, Ganz DA, et al. Inpatient fall prevention programs as a patient safety strategy: a systematic review. Ann Intern Med 2013;158: 390–6.
7. de Vries OJ, Peeters GM, Elders PJ, et al. Multifactorial intervention to reduce falls in older people at high risk of recurrent falls: a randomized controlled trial. Arch Intern Med 2010;170:1110–7.
8. Haines TP, Bennell KL, Osborne RH, et al. Effectiveness of targeted falls prevention programme in subacute hospital setting: randomised controlled trial. BMJ 2004;328:676.
9. Dykes PC, Carroll DL, Hurley A, et al. Fall prevention in acute care hospitals: a randomized trial. JAMA 2010;304:1912–8.
10. Stevens JA, Corso PS, Finkelstein EA, et al. The costs of fatal and non-fatal falls among older adults. Inj Prev 2006;12:290–5.
11. Services DoHaHSCfMM. Hospital-acquired condition (HAC) in acute inpatient payment system (IPPS) hospitals. Available at: http://www.cms.gov/Medicare/Medicare-Fee-for-Service-Payment/HospitalAcqCond/Downloads/HACFactsheet.pdf. Accessed March 12, 2014.
12. Kurtz S, Ong K, Lau E, et al. Projections of primary and revision hip and knee arthroplasty in the United States from 2005 to 2030. J Bone Joint Surg Am 2007;89:780–5.
13. Vetter TR, Ivankova NV, Goeddel LA, et al. An analysis of methodologies that can be used to validate if a perioperative surgical home improves the patient-centeredness, evidence-based practice, quality, safety, and value of patient care. Anesthesiology 2013;119:1261–74.
14. Choi M, Hector M. Effectiveness of intervention programs in preventing falls: a systematic review of recent 10 years and meta-analysis. J Am Med Dir Assoc 2012;13:188.e13–21.
15. Galbraith JG, Butler JS, Memon AR, et al. Cost analysis of a falls-prevention program in an orthopaedic setting. Clin Orthop Relat Res 2011;469:3462–8.
16. DiBardino D, Cohen ER, Didwania A. Meta-analysis: multidisciplinary fall prevention strategies in the acute care inpatient population. J Hosp Med 2012;7: 497–503.

17. The Joint Commission. Standards FAQ Details. Fall Reduction Program – NPSG – Goal 9-09.02.01. Available at: http://www.jointcommission.org/mobile/standards_information/jcfaqdetails.aspx?StandardsFAQId=201&StandardsFAQ Chapterld=77. Accessed April 11, 2014.
18. Ackerman DB, Trousdale RT, Bieber P, et al. Postoperative patient falls on an orthopedic inpatient unit. J Arthroplasty 2010;25:10–4.
19. Mandl LA, Lyman S, Quinlan P, et al. Falls among patients who had elective orthopaedic surgery: a decade of experience from a musculoskeletal specialty hospital. J Orthop Sports Phys Ther 2013;43:91–6.
20. Memtsoudis SG, Dy CJ, Ma Y, et al. In-hospital patient falls after total joint arthroplasty: incidence, demographics, and risk factors in the United States. J Arthroplasty 2012;27:823–8.e1.
21. Ilfeld BM, Duke KB, Donohue MC. The association between lower extremity continuous peripheral nerve blocks and patient falls after knee and hip arthroplasty. Anesth Analg 2010;111:1552–4.
22. Wasserstein D, Farlinger C, Brull R, et al. Advanced age, obesity and continuous femoral nerve blockade are independent risk factors for inpatient falls after primary total knee arthroplasty. J Arthroplasty 2013;28:1121–4.
23. Johnson RL, Kopp SL, Hebl JR, et al. Falls and major orthopaedic surgery with peripheral nerve blockade: a systematic review and meta-analysis. Br J Anaesth 2013;110:518–28.
24. Muraskin SI, Conrad B, Zheng N, et al. Falls associated with lower-extremity-nerve blocks: a pilot investigation of mechanisms. Reg Anesth Pain Med 2007;32:67–72.
25. Memtsoudis SG, Danninger T, Rasul R, et al. Inpatient falls after total knee arthroplasty: the role of anesthesia type and peripheral nerve blocks. Anesthesiology 2014;120:551–63.
26. Mudumbai SC, Kim TE, Howard SK, et al. Continuous adductor canal blocks are superior to continuous femoral nerve blocks in promoting early ambulation after TKA. Clin Orthop Relat Res 2014;472:1377–83.
27. Kim DH, Lin Y, Goytizolo EA, et al. Adductor canal block versus femoral nerve block for total knee arthroplasty: a prospective, randomized, controlled trial. Anesthesiology 2014;120:540–50.
28. Lohse GR, Leopold SS, Theiler S, et al. Systems-based safety intervention: reducing falls with injury and total falls on an orthopaedic ward. J Bone Joint Surg Am 2012;94:1217–22.
29. Bauer M, Wang L, Onibonoje OK, et al. Continuous femoral nerve blocks: decreasing local anesthetic concentration to minimize quadriceps femoris weakness. Anesthesiology 2012;116:665–72.
30. Ilfeld BM, Moeller LK, Mariano ER, et al. Continuous peripheral nerve blocks: is local anesthetic dose the only factor, or do concentration and volume influence infusion effects as well? Anesthesiology 2010;112:347–54.
31. Cui Q, Schapiro LH, Kinney MC, et al. Reducing costly falls of total knee replacement patients. Am J Med Qual 2013;28:335–8.
32. Hempel S, Newberry S, Wang Z, et al. Hospital fall prevention: a systematic review of implementation, components, adherence, and effectiveness. J Am Geriatr Soc 2013;61:483–94.
33. Stenvall M, Olofsson B, Lundstrom M, et al. A multidisciplinary, multifactorial intervention program reduces postoperative falls and injuries after femoral neck fracture. Osteoporos Int 2007;18:167–75.

34. Oliver D, Daly F, Martin FC, et al. Risk factors and risk assessment tools for falls in hospital in-patients: a systematic review. Age Ageing 2004;33:122–30.
35. Weinberg J, Proske D, Szerszen A, et al. An inpatient fall prevention initiative in a tertiary care hospital. Jt Comm J Qual Patient Saf 2011;37:317–25.
36. Haines TP, Hill AM, Hill KD, et al. Patient education to prevent falls among older hospital inpatients: a randomized controlled trial. Arch Intern Med 2011;171: 516–24.
37. Clarke HD, Timm VL, Goldberg BR, et al. Preoperative patient education reduces in-hospital falls after total knee arthroplasty. Clin Orthop Relat Res 2012;470: 244–9.
38. Mayo NE, Gloutney L, Levy AR. A randomized trial of identification bracelets to prevent falls among patients in a rehabilitation hospital. Arch Phys Med Rehabil 1994;75:1302–8.
39. Anderson O, Boshier PR, Hanna GB. Interventions designed to prevent healthcare bed-related injuries in patients. Cochrane Database Syst Rev 2012;(1):CD008931.
40. Shorr RI, Chandler AM, Mion LC, et al. Effects of an intervention to increase bed alarm use to prevent falls in hospitalized patients: a cluster randomized trial. Ann Intern Med 2012;157:692–9.
41. Innes EM. Maintaining fall prevention. QRB Qual Rev Bull 1985;11:217–21.
42. Ward A, Candela L, Mahoney J. Developing a unit-specific falls reduction program. J Healthc Qual 2004;26:36–40.
43. Dacenko-Grawe L, Holm K. Evidence-based practice: a falls prevention program that continues to work. Medsurg Nurs 2008;17:223–7, 235.

Optimizing Perioperative Management of Total Joint Arthroplasty

Rebecca L. Johnson, MD*, Sandra L. Kopp, MD

KEYWORDS

- Clinical pathways • Critical pathways • Perioperative care • Arthroplasty
- Replacement • Anesthesia • Conduction

KEY POINTS

- Total hip and knee arthroplasties are among the most common surgical procedures, using more Medicare procedural expenditures than any other surgery type.
- Optimizing patient status preoperatively and maximizing intraoperative management tactics to minimize postoperative complications may improve outcomes for total joint arthroplasty.
- Effective clinical pathways for total joint arthroplasty involve a multidisciplinary team that links evidence to practice and balances cost with local experience, outcomes, and access to resources, with the goal of efficient perioperative management.
- Clinical pathways for total joint arthroplasty require critical evaluation allowing for revision in light of outcomes and surgical and anesthesia practice changes.

INTRODUCTION

Total hip and knee arthroplasties are among the most common major surgical procedures performed within the United States.[1] Total joint arthroplasties are efficacious and cost-effective interventions linked to improving health-related quality of life and functional status of patients.[2–4] This comprehensive review of perioperative management of joint surgery explores:

- Trends in primary and revision joint arthroplasties
- Cost-effectiveness of clinical pathways
- Controversies in preoperative patient optimization for total joint arthroplasties
- Methods to maximize perioperative care for total joint arthroplasty

Financial Support: Mayo Clinic Foundation for Medical Education and Research.
Financial Disclosure: The authors have no financial interests or potential conflicts of interest.
Department of Anesthesiology, College of Medicine, Mayo Clinic, 200 First Street, Southwest, Rochester, MN 55905, USA
* Corresponding author.
E-mail address: johnson.rebecca1@mayo.edu

This review focuses on total knee arthroplasty (TKA) and total hip arthroplasty (THA), as these surgeries are associated with more pain and mobility restrictions than non–weight-bearing total joint arthroplasties.

Trends in Primary and Revision Total Knee and Total Hip Arthroplasty

Unlike countries with national registries, the number of total joint arthroplasties performed in the United States is not easily attainable, leaving projections to rely on representative surveys of hospital discharge records and Medicare administrative data.[2,5] Primary and revision total joint arthroplasties are projected to dramatically increase in the next 2 decades.[2,6,7] Primary THA will increase by 174% (572,000 surgeries by 2030), whereas primary TKA will increase by a staggering 673% to 3.48 million procedures (**Fig. 1**).[7] It is possible that this rapid increase in primary TKA and THA will lead to doubling in revision surgeries for knee replacement and for hip replacement by 2015 and 2026, respectively.

TKA is cost effective with reproducible positive outcomes including pain relief and improved functional status in patients with end-stage osteoarthritis compared with nonoperative management.[4] Losina and colleagues[4] found that even in low-volume hospitals, having a TKA was more cost effective in the long run than no surgery; this was true even among the highest-risk populations. Primary TKA, at a cost of $9 billion per year, may significantly increase future health care spending. If predictions are true and costs escalate further, the economic impact on hospitals from primary and revision total joint arthroplasty will be tremendous, considering Medicare reimbursements based on cost average only 32% to 38% per procedure.[8] Currently, total joint replacement represents the single greatest Medicare procedural disbursement. Therefore, changes in perioperative management that are designed to decrease or contain costs will continue to have a significant impact on US health care economics.[9,10] Clinical

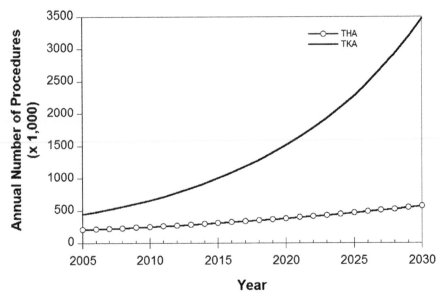

Fig. 1. The projected numbers of primary total joint arthroplasty in the United States from 2005 to 2030. (*From* Kurtz S, Ong K, Lau E, et al. Projections of primary and revision hip and knee arthroplasty in the United States from 2005 to 2030. J Bone Joint Surg Am 2007;89:783; with permission.)

pathways for total joint arthroplasty have been found to be effective in reducing total hospital costs and have positively impacted hospital length-of-stay by reducing provider variability.[9,11,12]

Deconstructing Clinical Pathways

Clinical pathways are tools created in the 1980s to organize care of well-defined groups of patients during well-defined periods of time.[13,14] These pathways are coordinated, evidenced-based, perioperative approaches specific to a surgical procedure. The goal is to modify preoperative preparation and standardize intraoperative and postoperative care.[15] No two clinical total joint pathways are the same, and there often is tremendous variability between institutions as a result of different patient populations, provider preferences, and resource availability.[16,17] This variability limits generalizability and prevents the development of a universal clinical pathway for specific orthopedic surgeries. Advantages and disadvantages to the use of clinical pathways for total joint arthroplasty are listed in **Box 1**.

The most effective clinical pathways are developed by a multidisciplinary group of providers (orthopedic surgeons, anesthesiologists, pharmacy, transfusion medicine, infectious disease, diabetes specialists, nursing, and rehabilitation therapists) who contribute ideas on standardization and reproducibility of care for patients undergoing total joint arthroplasty. Barbieri and colleagues[13] performed the largest systematic review and meta-analysis of clinical pathways for joint replacement surgery, analyzing 22 studies with 6316 patients. This review concluded that implementation of clinical pathways for joint replacement results in reduced postoperative complications (eg, infection and thromboembolism) and improved quality compared to standard care.

Effective clinical pathways for total joint arthroplasty link evidence to individual practices and balance costs with local experience, outcomes, and access to resources to provide responsible perioperative management. Clinical pathways are dynamic processes and should be revised in a timely manner based on emerging research. The

---

Box 1
Advantages and disadvantages of clinical pathways for total joint arthroplasty

Advantages

- Is a platform for coordinated care between departments and across patient care units

- Standardizes the process of patient care and reduces provider variability

- Decreases time-to-discharge readiness, which controls hospital costs by mainly reducing hospital length-of-stay

- Promotes practice change that emphasizes patient outcomes and cost containment

- Serves as a marketing tool with the public or third-party payers

Disadvantages

- Variables of clinical pathways differ between institutions (based on unique preferences and outcomes of the participating hospitals) making clinical comparisons of outcomes difficult across hospitals.

- Scientific rigor of clinical outcomes from clinical pathways is lacking (outcomes are analyzed retrospectively compared with historical controls or through audits).

- Scientific journals rarely publish outcomes data from clinical pathways leaving a void in formal guidelines or recommendations and preventing creation of a universal clinical pathway.

most consistent components of clinical pathways with major impact on improved perioperative outcomes in orthopedic patients are (1) implementing clinical pathways designed to include multimodal analgesia with regional anesthesia,[16–21] (2) the use of tranexamic acid to reduce blood loss in total joint arthroplasty,[22–29] and (3) preconditioning followed by participation in early and accelerated rehabilitation programs to prevent postoperative complications related to immobility.[30,31]

Multimodal analgesia and peripheral nerve blockade or local infiltration analgesia

Multimodal analgesia is a term that describes pain management, using both pharmacologic and nonpharmacologic techniques, which aims to maximize the positive aspects of treatment while limiting side effects.[21] Historically, perioperative pain control regimens for major orthopedic surgery utilized solely parenteral opioids. Patients often experienced opioid-related side effects (eg, sedation, nausea, vomiting, pruritus, ileus, urinary retention), which drastically impacted the rehabilitation process and hospital discharge readiness.[20,21,32,33] Because many of the negative side effects of analgesic therapy are opioid-related (and dose dependent), limiting perioperative opioid use is a major goal of multimodal analgesia. The most recent American Society of Anesthesiologists Task Force on Acute Pain Management[34] recommends the use of 2 or more analgesic modalities with different mechanisms of action that will provide analgesia while limiting side effects and adverse events. These expert guidelines have purposely allowed for broad interpretation. Hence, much debate exists across institutions as to which clinical pathway provides the ideal multimodal analgesic plan with the most value. Current use of clinical pathways with comprehensive, preemptive multimodal analgesia incorporating the use of regional anesthesia has been found to lower opioid requirements, minimize opioid-related side effects and complications, and reduce hospital length-of-stay after THA and TKA.[18,19,33]

Peripheral nerve blockade has become the gold standard for postoperative analgesia after THA and TKA.[18,19] Both single-injection[35–39] and continuous[40–46] peripheral nerve block techniques are proven to reduce perioperative complications, reduce hospital length-of-stay, conserve hospital resources, and enhance patient satisfaction. One potential disadvantage of common lower extremity peripheral nerve catheters is that patients often experience muscle weakness and restricted mobility. Some evidence suggests that this muscle weakness may increase the patient's risk of an in-hospital fall.[47–49] Reassuringly, a recent large retrospective study by Memtsoudis and colleagues[50] and a systematic review and meta-analysis by Johnson and colleagues[51] failed to reproduce previous reports[47,49,52] linking peripheral nerve blockade to increased fall risk. Regardless, many institutions have proactively started moving away from femoral nerve blocks as management options for TKA and have begun using peripheral nerve blocks promising less quadriceps weakness (adductor canal blockade). Randomized controlled trials comparing femoral nerve blockade with adductor canal blockade, in the context of an established multimodal analgesic pathway, have shown that when distal femoral block techniques are used, quadriceps weakness may be lessened without significant increases in postoperative pain.[53–56]

Unfortunately, long-term outcome studies examining preemptive oral medications such as nonsteroidal anti-inflammatory medications, acetaminophen, and low-dose opioids in isolation from peripheral nerve blockade do not exist. Currently, it is unknown if peripheral nerve blockade is a necessary component of clinical pathways or whether it is the collective multimodal approach that is of most benefit. Thus, clinical pathways are emerging using multimodal analgesia incorporating periarticular infiltration with long-acting local anesthesia and adjunct mixtures or ultra–long-acting liposomal bound local anesthesia injected into the wound at the time of surgery as alternatives to conventional peripheral nerve blockade.[57–59] At this time, some practices continue to use multimodal analgesia with peripheral nerve blockade, others have transitioned to premedications with local anesthetic periarticular infiltration, and still others use a combination of techniques and medications based on individual provider experiences and local resource availability. A selection of different options for controlling perioperative pain is included in **Box 2**.

Box 2
Multimodal analgesia options for controlling perioperative pain

Preoperative
Multimodal oral analgesia options
  Acetaminophen
  Oxycodone immediate or sustained release
  Celecoxib
  Gabapentin
Intraoperative
Regional analgesia options
  Total knee arthroplasty options
    Femoral block/catheter
    Sciatic block/catheter
    Adductor canal block/catheter
    Periarticular local anesthesia infiltration
    Epidural catheter
    Intrathecal opioids
  Total hip arthroplasty options
    Posterior lumbar plexus block/catheter
    Fascia Iliaca block/catheter
    Periarticular local anesthesia infiltration
    Epidural catheter
    Intrathecal opioids
Postoperative
Multimodal analgesia options
  Acetaminophen
  Low-dose opioid (eg, oxycodone)
  Ketorolac
  Tramadol
  Ketamine
  Lidocaine
  Dexamethasone
  Clonidine
  Peripheral nerve catheter with local anesthesia infusion

Preventing the transition from acute to chronic pain

It is unknown whether the immediate postoperative benefits from multimodal analgesia pathways with regional anesthesia affect long-term outcomes, such as the development of persistent postoperative pain after total joint arthroplasty. Surprisingly, despite receiving a brand new joint, only 80% to 85% of patients undergoing TKA report satisfaction with their surgery.[60] Jacobs and Christensen[61] found that patients who are dissatisfied 2 and 5 years after TKA are more likely to have higher immediate postoperative pain scores and fail to experience improvements in passive flexion or functional scores compared with their preoperative status. In fact, this study also indicates that poor pain relief at short-term to midterm follow-up alone can be predictive of patient dissatisfaction.

Persistent postoperative pain, (pain lasting >3 months), is common and can affect 10% to 50% of certain surgical populations.[62] However, persistent pain after total joint arthroplasty is often underappreciated.[63] Wylde and colleagues[63] report that 44% of TKA patients and 27% of THA patients have persistent postsurgical pain. This pain is labeled as severe to extreme pain in 15% after TKA and 1% after THA. Risk factors for persistent pain include duration of preoperative pain, female sex, depression, and presence of pain in more than one body location.[63–65] Although these high-risk populations have been identified, future research is necessary to determine if there are any interventions to specifically reduce rates of chronic pain in these subpopulations. Brander and colleagues[66] found presurgical knee pain of more than a year in duration to be a significant risk factor for chronic pain; however, the strongest predictor for persistent pain after TKA reported in this study was the intensity of pain in the first week after surgery. Similarly, Nikolajsen and colleagues[64] in their study of THA report that persistent postsurgical pain was dependent on the recalled intensity of early postoperative pain rather than the intensity of preoperative pain levels.

Some suggest that pain is on a continuum and that interventions targeting acute postoperative pain severity could prevent the development of chronic pain. Therefore, it is critically important that clinical pathways use the best evidence-based modalities for reducing acute postoperative pain.

Limiting blood transfusions with tranexamic acid

Total joint arthroplasties can result in significant blood loss (mean of 1500 mL) not uncommonly necessitating blood transfusion.[67] However, many institutions have developed clinical pathways that incorporate blood management strategies to limit allogenic blood transfusion because of concerns of posttransfusion complications, including increased infection rates.[68–71] Blood transfusions have been shown to induce transfusion-related immunomodulation, which has been linked to infection and even tumor recurrence.[72] In fact, allogenic blood transfusion has been associated with worsening mortality,[73] overall wound infections,[69,74] and prolonged hospital stay.[75] Strategies that reduce intraoperative and postoperative bleeding should be essential components of clinical pathways to optimize outcomes after total joint arthroplasties.

Treating anemia in the preoperative period Preoperative anemia (hemoglobin <12 g/dL for females and <13 g/dL for males) is highly prevalent among surgical patients.[76] Perioperative anemia is associated with higher rates of blood transfusion, postoperative infection, poor physical function, and rehabilitation as well as increased hospital stays and mortality.[76–78] Iron deficiency anemia and anemia of chronic disease are commonly found among orthopedic surgical populations. Surgical bleeding further depletes iron stores, making correction of anemia preoperatively with supplemental oral or intravenous iron an important strategy for reducing postoperative anemia and need for allogenic blood transfusion.[77,79] Clinical care pathways should incorporate preoperative investigations of anemia, and correction of reversible causes should be considered before elective surgery.

Tranexamic acid Antifibrinolytic medications such as tranexamic acid (TXA), aprotinin, and aminocaproic acid have been used effectively for minimizing perioperative blood loss and massive transfusion in obstetrics,[80] trauma surgery,[81,82] and cardiac surgery.[83,84] Within orthopedic surgery, TXA has been the most studied. TXA, a synthetic amino acid lysine analog, inhibits plasminogen activation, ultimately reducing fibrinolysis of existing thrombi. Evidence is mounting to support widespread use for TXA for reducing perioperative blood loss and allogenic transfusion after THA[26,85] and TKA.[22,23,25–27] Additionally, Gillette and colleagues[24] discovered routine use of TXA is cost effective, as the pharmacy costs of TXA administration can be more than offset by lower hospital total costs related to transfusion. Opponents to TXA use mention concerns that TXA may elevate risk for blood clotting and cite that orthopedic patients are already at elevated risk for thromboembolism based on age and immobility factors. Although no individual study has sufficient power to prove safety against low incidence complications such as thromboembolism, recent meta-analyses investigating efficacy and safety of TXA in TKA[27] and THA[29] have shown no increased risks of complications compared with no TXA use. Moreover, Whiting and coinvestigators,[28] in a recent retrospective study, did not find TXA to be associated with any increased thromboembolism events within 30 days of surgery even among patients at higher risk for such complications (eg, ASA III and IV patients). The protocol for TXA use at Whiting's institution, which performs more than 3000 elective hip and knee replacements annually, includes providing 1 g of intravenous TXA before incision (administered along with prophylactic antibiotics) and adding a second dose of 1 g at initiation of wound closure (timed based on the drug's 2 hour half-life).[86] This practice does provide for a multiple-dose strategy, with a dosing regimen of 10 mg to 20 mg/kg per dose, which has been proven more effective than using single bolus administration.[87]

Early and accelerated rehabilitation

Clinical pathways for total joint arthroplasty that focus on patient preconditioning (eg, fitness programs before surgery) followed by early and accelerated rehabilitation postoperatively have proven more effective for reducing costs by shortening hospital length-of-stay and achieving faster functional outcomes such as distance ambulated compared with delayed rehabilitation programs.[30,31] Additional factors that are critical to patient participation in accelerated rehabilitation programs include controlling pain and providing emotional support.[88,89] Patient motivation is likely the single most important key for success after total joint arthroplasty. Unfortunately, motivation is unlikely influenced by anesthesiologists. However, providing adequate analgesia in the perioperative period can and should continue to be our primary goal, as failures in pain management can impede the initiation of early physical therapy leaving even the most motivated of patients vulnerable to postoperative complications.

Current Controversies in Preoperative Optimization

Today's clinical pathways should incorporate ways to optimize patient's health preoperatively, especially as our patients become more medically complex. A recent analysis of Medicare administrative data from 1991 to 2010 showed that (1) TKA procedures are increasing, (2) patients are leaving the hospital sooner, and (3) patients are more likely to be discharged home with outpatient rehabilitation rather than to skilled nursing facilities.[2] As a result of this observed reduction in length-of-stay and discharge to dispositions with less supervision, there was an accompanying increase in readmission rates for postoperative complications over the last decade. This information suggests that there are limits to the extent that hospital length-of-stay can and should be reduced and leads us to question why we are trying to control costs by pushing to contain only direct, hospital-related expenses.

Currently, the most common complication and reason for readmission after both primary and revision joint arthroplasty is infection.[2,5] Deep prosthetic joint infections after primary total joint arthroplasty are serious postoperative complications reported to occur as frequently as 0.51% to 2% among high-risk patients.[90–95] According to Medicare data, the rate of periprosthetic infections within the first 2 years after TKA is 1.55%. Considering these high-risk complications are likely to increase with increasing surgical volumes, prevention strategies must be used. With the introduction of the Perioperative Surgical Home model,[96–98] anesthesiology is evolving into the practice of perioperative medicine, and anesthesiologists may find themselves in a unique position to focus on perioperative factors that may help prevent these devastating postoperative infections. Patient-, surgical-, or anesthesia-related variables associated with all infections (including but not specific to periprosthetic infection) that may be modifiable are provided in **Box 3**.

Malnutrition and morbid obesity

Morbid obesity (body mass index >40 kg/m^2) and malnutrition are both independent risk factors for postoperative complications, including surgical site infections, after both THA[90] and TKA.[91] Not uncommonly, despite their size, these patients can have a poor nutritional status. Drs Garvin and Konigsberg, instructors at The American Academy of Orthopedic Surgeons, suggest that patients should be screened preoperatively for malnutrition (a transferrin level of <200 mg/dL, an albumin level <3.5 g/dL, or a total lymphocyte count of <1500 cells/mm^3) and referred for nutritional counseling before major orthopedic surgery.[94] For those without serologic evidence of poor nutrition, weight reduction, including bariatric surgery, has also been strongly advocated

---

Box 3
Potential modifiable patient-, surgical-, or anesthesia-related variables associated with infections

Patient characteristics

- Diabetes mellitus
- Body mass index ≥35 kg/m^2
- Smoking
- Alcoholism
- Urinary tract infection
- Poor nutritional status

Surgical or anesthesia factors

- Extended operating time (>2.5 hours)
- Blood transfusion
- Primary anesthesia type

for patients with morbid obesity as potential first-line interventions before offering orthopedic surgery as strategies for reducing surgical site infection.[92–94]

Tobacco abuse

Tobacco abuse has also been associated with increased rates of surgical site infections.[99,100] Nicotine-mediated vasoconstriction is considered a primary cause of decreased blood flow to tissues resulting in deoxygenation and tissue devitalization.[101] Moreover, smoking has been linked to delayed bone healing, which may contribute to implant loosening. It is not surprising that, for these reasons, tobacco use likely affects overall prosthesis survival with studies indicating that smokers are more likely to require revision TKA[100] and THA[99] compared with nonsmokers. Perhaps, smoking cessation counseling and participation in programs designed to quit smoking should be given stronger consideration before offering elective total joint arthroplasty.

Glycemic control

More than 8% of patients undergoing total joint arthroplasty in the United States have diabetes mellitus (DM).[102] Diabetic patients, even under good control, are at high risk for common surgical and systemic complications including surgical site infection and prolonged hospital stays.[90,91,102] In addition, poorly controlled DM independently elevates the risk of postoperative morbidity and mortality compared with controlled DM.[103] In a large retrospective study of nearly 1 million patients in the Nationwide Inpatient Sample, Marchant and colleagues[103] found patients with uncontrolled DM compared with those with controlled DM regardless of diabetes subtype (type I or II DM) were likely to stay in the hospital longer and suffer higher rates of death and major morbidities (eg, infection, stroke, hemorrhage). The American Diabetes Association recommends hemoglobin A1c values should be less than 7.0% for most patients to reduce the risk of microvascular disease.[104] This information leads us to recommend that intraoperative glycemic control initiatives should be part of future clinical pathways for total joint arthroplasty, and we as perioperative physicians may need to question pursuits of elective total joint arthroplasty on those with poorly controlled DM.

Patient education

Another important component of perioperative total joint arthroplasty pathways that is often overlooked is patient education. Surgery is a stressful process. Preoperative education in total joint arthroplasty has been proposed as a method to reduce anxiety in the preoperative period.[105,106] However, the same authors acknowledge that this positive effect on preoperative anxiety and knowledge level has yet to be linked to changes in postoperative outcomes including pain, range-of-motion, function, or length-of-hospitalization. Although patients are often educated, it appears that not always is the education effective. This may be especially true when considering patient expectations regarding tolerable levels of pain in the postoperative period.

Interestingly, some patients will perceive and complain of unacceptable pain postoperatively, despite normal clinical examination and radiographic evidence of acceptable outcomes. This finding has led many to question whether the perioperative team is educating the patient properly about the psychological factors that can alter postoperative outcomes. In a prospective, observational study of patients undergoing TKA, Brander and colleagues[66] identified normal pain recovery patterns and factors associated with high postoperative pain reports. As expected, pain was noted to be significant (Visual Analog Scale >40) on a 0 to 100 scale preoperatively in 72.3% of patients and despite surgical intervention was still significant in 13.1% of patients at 12 months.[66] Preoperative depression and anxiety symptoms and greater preoperative pain were all independent and additive predictors for significant pain at 12 months.

Preoperative education designed to answer the common question "how long will pain last after surgery?" may help frame postoperative expectations for patients. Evidence suggests that informing your patient that pain after TKA should reduce to half of your preoperative value by 3 months after surgery and may never be completely abolished sets more realistic expectations of pain outcomes and makes the surgical process more transparent.

Aggressive treatment of postoperative pain is not without potential consequences. In 2001, the Joint Commission on Accreditation of Healthcare Organizations introduced standards that mandated pain management become an integral component of hospital patient care. Implementation of hospital-wide pain management protocols that based treatment algorithms on patient self-reports became the norm. Patients were educated that pain was a "fifth vital sign," and analgesic management was guided poorly by these subjective methods of pain assessment. Vila and colleagues[107] showed that although patient satisfaction improved as a result of the adoption of Joint Commission on Accreditation of Healthcare Organizations standards, their hospital experienced a more than 2-fold increase in incidence of opioid-induced respiratory depression. In this study, more than 94% of events were preceded by a decreased level of consciousness. Perhaps development of pain management algorithms that incorporate both subjective ratings of pain along with objective assessments of consciousness are necessary and may provide a greater margin of safety. Without question, future research to investigate how to reduce anxiety while also showing a safe reduction in postoperative pain or improvements in functional outcomes is needed.

FUTURE CONSIDERATIONS/SUMMARY

Defining optimal perioperative care for total joint arthroplasty is difficult, as "successful outcomes" reflects the agendas and values of many stakeholders (eg, patients, physicians, and institutions). Patients may report high satisfaction if they have no pain during the perioperative period. However, pain-free surgery is an unrealistic and perhaps even deadly goal. On the opposite end of the spectrum, early hospital discharge without adequate acute pain management leads to readmission and postoperative complications along with high rates of patient dissatisfaction. This conflict in outcome prioritization has led to a movement that future clinical trials should consider more than just acute pain management.[108,109] The Initiative on Methods, Measurements, and Pain Assessment in Clinical Trials (IMMPACT) recommends that not only pain outcomes but also physical and emotional functioning, participant ratings of improvement and satisfaction with treatment, symptoms and adverse outcomes, and participant disposition be considered. In other words, there may be little role to implementing treatments that provide only evidence of improvements in the pain outcome domain alone moving forward; instead, evidence that interventions show lasting benefit for patients by preventing chronic pain development or producing functional improvements without adverse outcomes may be required.

This comprehensive review of perioperative management of joint surgery examined the use of clinical pathways for TKA and THA, discussed many controversial issues of major orthopedic surgery, and provided some suggestions of how anesthesiologists may serve as the ideal perioperative medicine experts for total joint arthroplasty.

REFERENCES

1. Finks JF, Osborne NH, Birkmeyer JD. Trends in hospital volume and operative mortality for high-risk surgery. N Engl J Med 2011;364:2128–37.

2. Cram P, Lu X, Kates SL, et al. Total knee arthroplasty volume, utilization, and outcomes among Medicare beneficiaries, 1991-2010. JAMA 2012;308:1227–36.
3. Larsen K, Hansen TB, Thomsen PB, et al. Cost-effectiveness of accelerated perioperative care and rehabilitation after total hip and knee arthroplasty. J Bone Joint Surg Am 2009;91:761–72.
4. Losina E, Walensky RP, Kessler CL, et al. Cost-effectiveness of total knee arthroplasty in the United States: patient risk and hospital volume. Arch Intern Med 2009;169:1113–21 [discussion: 1121–2].
5. Bozic KJ, Kurtz SM, Lau E, et al. The epidemiology of revision total knee arthroplasty in the United States. Clin Orthop Relat Res 2010;468:45–51.
6. Kurtz S, Mowat F, Ong K, et al. Prevalence of primary and revision total hip and knee arthroplasty in the United States from 1990 through 2002. J Bone Joint Surg Am 2005;87:1487–97.
7. Kurtz S, Ong K, Lau E, et al. Projections of primary and revision hip and knee arthroplasty in the United States from 2005 to 2030. J Bone Joint Surg Am 2007;89:780–5.
8. Ong KL, Mowat FS, Chan N, et al. Economic burden of revision hip and knee arthroplasty in Medicare enrollees. Clin Orthop Relat Res 2006;446:22–8.
9. Duncan CM, Hall Long K, Warner DO, et al. The economic implications of a multimodal analgesic regimen for patients undergoing major orthopedic surgery: a comparative study of direct costs. Reg Anesth Pain Med 2009;34:301–7.
10. Meyers SJ, Reuben JD, Cox DD, et al. Inpatient cost of primary total joint arthroplasty. J Arthroplasty 1996;11:281–5.
11. Ho DM, Huo MH. Are critical pathways and implant standardization programs effective in reducing costs in total knee replacement operations? J Am Coll Surg 2007;205:97–100.
12. Macario A, Horne M, Goodman S, et al. The effect of a perioperative clinical pathway for knee replacement surgery on hospital costs. Anesth Analg 1998; 86:978–84.
13. Barbieri A, Vanhaecht K, Van Herck P, et al. Effects of clinical pathways in the joint replacement: a meta-analysis. BMC Med 2009;7:32.
14. Panella M, Marchisio S, Di Stanislao F. Reducing clinical variations with clinical pathways: do pathways work? Int J Qual Health Care 2003;15:509–21.
15. Carli F, Kehlet H, Baldini G, et al. Evidence basis for regional anesthesia in multidisciplinary fast-track surgical care pathways. Reg Anesth Pain Med 2011;36: 63–72.
16. Johnson RL, Duncan CM, Hebl JR. Clinical pathways for total joint arthroplasty: essential components for success. Adv Anesth 2011;29:149–71.
17. Williams BA, Kentor MI. Clinical pathways and the anesthesiologist. Curr Anesthesiol Rep 2000;2000:418–24.
18. Hebl JR, Dilger JA, Byer DE, et al. A pre-emptive multimodal pathway featuring peripheral nerve block improves perioperative outcomes after major orthopedic surgery. Reg Anesth Pain Med 2008;33:510–7.
19. Hebl JR, Kopp SL, Ali MH, et al. A comprehensive anesthesia protocol that emphasizes peripheral nerve blockade for total knee and total hip arthroplasty. J Bone Joint Surg Am 2005;87(Suppl 2):63–70.
20. Horlocker TT. Pain management in total joint arthroplasty: a historical review. Orthopedics 2010;33:14–9.
21. Horlocker TT, Kopp SL, Pagnano MW, et al. Analgesia for total hip and knee arthroplasty: a multimodal pathway featuring peripheral nerve block. J Am Acad Orthop Surg 2006;14:126–35.

22. Aguilera X, Martinez-Zapata MJ, Bosch A, et al. Efficacy and safety of fibrin glue and tranexamic acid to prevent postoperative blood loss in total knee arthroplasty: a randomized controlled clinical trial. J Bone Joint Surg Am 2013;95:2001–7.

23. Cid J, Lozano M. Tranexamic acid reduces allogeneic red cell transfusions in patients undergoing total knee arthroplasty: results of a meta-analysis of randomized controlled trials. Transfusion 2005;45:1302–7.

24. Gillette BP, Maradit Kremers H, Duncan CM, et al. Economic impact of tranexamic acid in healthy patients undergoing primary total hip and knee arthroplasty. J Arthroplasty 2013;28:137–9.

25. Kelley TC, Tucker KK, Adams MJ, et al. Use of tranexamic acid results in decreased blood loss and decreased transfusions in patients undergoing staged bilateral total knee arthroplasty. Transfusion 2014;54:26–30.

26. Oremus K, Sostaric S, Trkulja V, et al. Influence of tranexamic acid on postoperative autologous blood retransfusion in primary total hip and knee arthroplasty: a randomized controlled trial. Transfusion 2014;54:31–41.

27. Tan J, Chen H, Liu Q, et al. A meta-analysis of the effectiveness and safety of using tranexamic acid in primary unilateral total knee arthroplasty. J Surg Res 2013;184:880–7.

28. Whiting DR, Gillette BP, Duncan C, et al. Preliminary results suggest tranexamic acid is safe and effective in arthroplasty patients with severe comorbidities. Clin Orthop Relat Res 2014;472:66–72.

29. Zhou XD, Tao LJ, Li J, et al. Do we really need tranexamic acid in total hip arthroplasty? A meta-analysis of nineteen randomized controlled trials. Arch Orthop Trauma Surg 2013;133:1017–27.

30. Munin MC, Rudy TE, Glynn NW, et al. Early inpatient rehabilitation after elective hip and knee arthroplasty. JAMA 1998;279:847–52.

31. Pour AE, Parvizi J, Sharkey PF, et al. Minimally invasive hip arthroplasty: what role does patient preconditioning play? J Bone Joint Surg Am 2007;89:1920–7.

32. Kehlet H, Dahl JB. The value of multimodal or balanced analgesia in postoperative pain treatment. Anesth Analg 1993;77:1048–56.

33. Parvizi J, Miller AG, Gandhi K. Multimodal pain management after total joint arthroplasty. J Bone Joint Surg Am 2011;93:1075–84.

34. American Society of Anesthesiologists Task Force on Acute PainManagement. Practice guidelines for acute pain management in the perioperative setting: an updated report by the American Society of Anesthesiologists Task Force on Acute Pain Management. Anesthesiology 2012;116:248–73.

35. Allen HW, Liu SS, Ware PD, et al. Peripheral nerve blocks improve analgesia after total knee replacement surgery. Anesth Analg 1998;87:93–7.

36. Biboulet P, Morau D, Aubas P, et al. Postoperative analgesia after total-hip arthroplasty: comparison of intravenous patient-controlled analgesia with morphine and single injection of femoral nerve or psoas compartment block. A prospective, randomized, double-blind study. Reg Anesth Pain Med 2004;29:102–9.

37. Szczukowski MJ Jr, Hines JA, Snell JA, et al. Femoral nerve block for total knee arthroplasty patients: a method to control postoperative pain. J Arthroplasty 2004;19:720–5.

38. Wang H, Boctor B, Verner J. The effect of single-injection femoral nerve block on rehabilitation and length of hospital stay after total knee replacement. Reg Anesth Pain Med 2002;27:139–44.

39. YaDeau JT, Cahill JB, Zawadsky MW, et al. The effects of femoral nerve blockade in conjunction with epidural analgesia after total knee arthroplasty. Anesth Analg 2005;101:891–5 table of contents.

40. Edwards ND, Wright EM. Continuous low-dose 3-in-1 nerve blockade for post-operative pain relief after total knee replacement. Anesth Analg 1992;75:265–7.
41. Ganapathy S, Wasserman RA, Watson JT, et al. Modified continuous femoral three-in-one block for postoperative pain after total knee arthroplasty. Anesth Analg 1999;89:1197–202.
42. Ilfeld BM, Ball ST, Gearen PF, et al. Ambulatory continuous posterior lumbar plexus nerve blocks after hip arthroplasty: a dual-center, randomized, triple-masked, placebo-controlled trial. Anesthesiology 2008;109:491–501.
43. Ilfeld BM, Le LT, Meyer RS, et al. Ambulatory continuous femoral nerve blocks decrease time to discharge readiness after tricompartment total knee arthro-plasty: a randomized, triple-masked, placebo-controlled study. Anesthesiology 2008;108:703–13.
44. Kaloul I, Guay J, Cote C, et al. The posterior lumbar plexus (psoas compart-ment) block and the three-in-one femoral nerve block provide similar postoper-ative analgesia after total knee replacement. Can J Anaesth 2004;51:45–51.
45. Siddiqui ZI, Cepeda MS, Denman W, et al. Continuous lumbar plexus block provides improved analgesia with fewer side effects compared with systemic opioids after hip arthroplasty: a randomized controlled trial. Reg Anesth Pain Med 2007;32:393–8.
46. Singelyn FJ, Deyaert M, Joris D, et al. Effects of intravenous patient-controlled analgesia with morphine, continuous epidural analgesia, and continuous three-in-one block on postoperative pain and knee rehabilitation after unilateral total knee arthroplasty. Anesth Analg 1998;87:88–92.
47. Ilfeld BM, Duke KB, Donohue MC. The association between lower extremity continuous peripheral nerve blocks and patient falls after knee and hip arthro-plasty. Anesth Analg 2010;111:1552–4.
48. Kandasami M, Kinninmonth AW, Sarungi M, et al. Femoral nerve block for total knee replacement - a word of caution. Knee 2009;16:98–100.
49. Sharma S, Iorio R, Specht LM, et al. Complications of femoral nerve block for total knee arthroplasty. Clin Orthop Relat Res 2010;468:135–40.
50. Memtsoudis SG, Danninger T, Rasul R, et al. Inpatient falls after total knee arthroplasty: the role of anesthesia type and peripheral nerve blocks. Anesthe-siology 2014;120:551–63.
51. Johnson RL, Kopp SL, Hebl JR, et al. Falls and major orthopaedic surgery with peripheral nerve blockade: a systematic review and meta-analysis. Br J Anaesth 2013;110:518–28.
52. Feibel RJ, Dervin GF, Kim PR, et al. Major complications associated with femoral nerve catheters for knee arthroplasty: a word of caution. J Arthroplasty 2009;24:132–7.
53. Jaeger P, Nielsen ZJ, Henningsen MH, et al. Adductor canal block versus femoral nerve block and quadriceps strength: a randomized, double-blind, pla-cebo-controlled, crossover study in healthy volunteers. Anesthesiology 2013;118:409–15.
54. Jaeger P, Zaric D, Fomsgaard JS, et al. Adductor canal block versus femoral nerve block for analgesia after total knee arthroplasty: a randomized, double-blind study. Reg Anesth Pain Med 2013;38:526–32.
55. Kim DH, Lin Y, Goytizolo EA, et al. Adductor canal block versus femoral nerve block for total knee arthroplasty: a prospective, randomized, controlled trial. Anesthesiology 2014;120:540–50.
56. Kwofie MK, Shastri UD, Gadsden JC, et al. The effects of ultrasound-guided adductor canal block versus femoral nerve block on quadriceps strength and

fall risk: a blinded, randomized trial of volunteers. Reg Anesth Pain Med 2013; 38:321–5.

57. Kerr DR, Kohan L. Local infiltration analgesia: a technique for the control of acute postoperative pain following knee and hip surgery: a case study of 325 patients. Acta Orthop 2008;79:174–83.

58. McCarthy D, Iohom G. Local infiltration analgesia for postoperative pain control following total hip arthroplasty: a systematic review. Anesthesiol Res Pract 2012; 2012:709531.

59. Parvataneni HK, Shah VP, Howard H, et al. Controlling pain after total hip and knee arthroplasty using a multimodal protocol with local periarticular injections: a prospective randomized study. J Arthroplasty 2007;22:33–8.

60. Scott CE, Howie CR, MacDonald D, et al. Predicting dissatisfaction following total knee replacement: a prospective study of 1217 patients. J Bone Joint Surg Br 2010;92:1253–8.

61. Jacobs CA, Christensen CP. Factors influencing patient satisfaction two to five years after primary total knee arthroplasty. J Arthroplasty 2014;29:1189–91.

62. Kehlet H, Jensen TS, Woolf CJ. Persistent postsurgical pain: risk factors and prevention. Lancet 2006;367:1618–25.

63. Wylde V, Hewlett S, Learmonth ID, et al. Persistent pain after joint replacement: prevalence, sensory qualities, and postoperative determinants. Pain 2011;152: 566–72.

64. Nikolajsen L, Brandsborg B, Lucht U, et al. Chronic pain following total hip arthroplasty: a nationwide questionnaire study. Acta Anaesthesiol Scand 2006;50:495–500.

65. Puolakka PA, Rorarius MG, Roviola M, et al. Persistent pain following knee arthroplasty. Eur J Anaesthesiol 2010;27:455–60.

66. Brander VA, Stulberg SD, Adams AD, et al. Predicting total knee replacement pain: a prospective, observational study. Clin Orthop Relat Res 2003;(416):27–36.

67. Sehat KR, Evans RL, Newman JH. Hidden blood loss following hip and knee arthroplasty. Correct management of blood loss should take hidden loss into account. J Bone Joint Surg Br 2004;86:561–5.

68. Duffy G, Neal KR. Differences in post-operative infection rates between patients receiving autologous and allogeneic blood transfusion: a meta-analysis of published randomized and nonrandomized studies. Transfus Med 1996;6:325–8.

69. Friedman R, Homering M, Holberg G, et al. Allogeneic blood transfusions and postoperative infections after total hip or knee arthroplasty. J Bone Joint Surg Am 2014;96:272–8.

70. Newman ET, Watters TS, Lewis JS, et al. Impact of perioperative allogeneic and autologous blood transfusion on acute wound infection following total knee and total hip arthroplasty. J Bone Joint Surg Am 2014;96:279–84.

71. Yates AJ Jr. The relative risk of infection from transfusions after arthroplasty: commentary on articles by Richard Friedman, MD, FRCSC, et al.: "Allogeneic blood transfusions and postoperative infections after total hip or knee arthroplasty" and Erik T. Newman, MD, et al.: "Impact of perioperative allogeneic and autologous blood transfusion on acute wound infection following total knee and total hip arthroplasty". J Bone Joint Surg Am 2014;96:e33.

72. Vamvakas EC, Blajchman MA. Transfusion-related immunomodulation (TRIM): an update. Blood Rev 2007;21:327–48.

73. Bierbaum BE, Callaghan JJ, Galante JO, et al. An analysis of blood management in patients having a total hip or knee arthroplasty. J Bone Joint Surg Am 1999;81:2–10.

74. Innerhofer P, Klingler A, Klimmer C, et al. Risk for postoperative infection after transfusion of white blood cell-filtered allogeneic or autologous blood components in orthopedic patients undergoing primary arthroplasty. Transfusion 2005;45: 103–10.

75. Weber EW, Slappendel R, Prins MH, et al. Perioperative blood transfusions and delayed wound healing after hip replacement surgery: effects on duration of hospitalization. Anesth Analg 2005;100:1416–21 table of contents.

76. Shander A, Knight K, Thurer R, et al. Prevalence and outcomes of anemia in surgery: a systematic review of the literature. Am J Med 2004;116(Suppl 7A): 58S–69S.

77. Goodnough LT, Shander A, Spivak JL, et al. Detection, evaluation, and management of anemia in the elective surgical patient. Anesth Analg 2005;101:1858–61.

78. Spahn DR. Anemia and patient blood management in hip and knee surgery: a systematic review of the literature. Anesthesiology 2010;113:482–95.

79. Cuenca J, Garcia-Erce JA, Martinez F, et al. Preoperative haematinics and transfusion protocol reduce the need for transfusion after total knee replacement. Int J Surg 2007;5:89–94.

80. Pham HP, Shaz BH. Update on massive transfusion. Br J Anaesth 2013; 111(Suppl 1):i71–82.

81. Morrison JJ, Dubose JJ, Rasmussen TE, et al. Military application of tranexamic acid in trauma emergency resuscitation (MATTERs) Study. Arch Surg 2012;147: 113–9.

82. Shakur H, Roberts I, Bautista R, et al. Effects of tranexamic acid on death, vascular occlusive events, and blood transfusion in trauma patients with significant haemorrhage (CRASH-2): a randomised, placebo-controlled trial. Lancet 2010;376:23–32.

83. Bokesch PM, Szabo G, Wojdyga R, et al. A phase 2 prospective, randomized, double-blind trial comparing the effects of tranexamic acid with ecallantide on blood loss from high-risk cardiac surgery with cardiopulmonary bypass (CONSERV-2 Trial). J Thorac Cardiovasc Surg 2012;143:1022–9.

84. Wang G, Xie G, Jiang T, et al. Tranexamic acid reduces blood loss after off-pump coronary surgery: a prospective, randomized, double-blind, placebo-controlled study. Anesth Analg 2012;115:239–43.

85. Sukeik M, Alshryda S, Haddad FS, et al. Systematic review and meta-analysis of the use of tranexamic acid in total hip replacement. J Bone Joint Surg Br 2011; 93:39–46.

86. Watts CD, Pagnano MW. Minimising blood loss and transfusion in contemporary hip and knee arthroplasty. J Bone Joint Surg Br 2012;94:8–10.

87. Maniar RN, Kumar G, Singhi T, et al. Most effective regimen of tranexamic acid in knee arthroplasty: a prospective randomized controlled study in 240 patients. Clin Orthop Relat Res 2012;470:2605–12.

88. Ranawat AS, Ranawat CS. Pain management and accelerated rehabilitation for total hip and total knee arthroplasty. J Arthroplasty 2007;22:12–5.

89. Ranawat CS, Ranawat AS, Mehta A. Total knee arthroplasty rehabilitation protocol: what makes the difference? J Arthroplasty 2003;18:27–30.

90. Dowsey MM, Choong PF. Obesity is a major risk factor for prosthetic infection after primary hip arthroplasty. Clin Orthop Relat Res 2008;466:153–8.

91. Dowsey MM, Choong PF. Obese diabetic patients are at substantial risk for deep infection after primary TKA. Clin Orthop Relat Res 2009;467:1577–81.

92. Jamsen E, Nevalainen P, Eskelinen A, et al. Obesity, diabetes, and preoperative hyperglycemia as predictors of periprosthetic joint infection: a single-center

analysis of 7181 primary hip and knee replacements for osteoarthritis. J Bone Joint Surg Am 2012;94:e101.

93. Malinzak RA, Ritter MA, Berend ME, et al. Morbidly obese, diabetic, younger, and unilateral joint arthroplasty patients have elevated total joint arthroplasty infection rates. J Arthroplasty 2009;24:84–8.

94. Garvin KL, Konigsberg BS. Infection following total knee arthroplasty: prevention and management. J Bone Joint Surg Am 2011;93:1167–75.

95. Namba RS, Inacio MC, Paxton EW. Risk factors associated with deep surgical site infections after primary total knee arthroplasty: an analysis of 56,216 knees. J Bone Joint Surg Am 2013;95:775–82.

96. Grocott MP, Pearse RM. Perioperative medicine: the future of anaesthesia? Br J Anaesth 2012;108:723–6.

97. Vetter TR, Goeddel LA, Boudreaux AM, et al. The perioperative surgical home: how can it make the case so everyone wins? BMC Anesthesiol 2013;13:6.

98. Vetter TR, Ivankova NV, Goeddel LA, et al. An analysis of methodologies that can be used to validate if a perioperative surgical home improves the patient-centeredness, evidence-based practice, quality, safety, and value of patient care. Anesthesiology 2013;119:1261–74.

99. Kapadia BH, Issa K, Pivec R, et al. Tobacco use may be associated with increased revision and complication rates following total hip arthroplasty. J Arthroplasty 2014;29:777–80.

100. Kapadia BH, Johnson AJ, Naziri Q, et al. Increased revision rates after total knee arthroplasty in patients who smoke. J Arthroplasty 2012;27:1690–5.e1.

101. Black CE, Huang N, Neligan PC, et al. Effect of nicotine on vasoconstrictor and vasodilator responses in human skin vasculature. Am J Physiol Regul Integr Comp Physiol 2001;281:R1097–104.

102. Bolognesi MP, Marchant MH Jr, Viens NA, et al. The impact of diabetes on perioperative patient outcomes after total hip and total knee arthroplasty in the United States. J Arthroplasty 2008;23:92–8.

103. Marchant MH Jr, Viens NA, Cook C, et al. The impact of glycemic control and diabetes mellitus on perioperative outcomes after total joint arthroplasty. J Bone Joint Surg Am 2009;91:1621–9.

104. American Diabetes Association. Standards of medical care in diabetes–2011. Diabetes Care 2011;34(Suppl 1):S11–61.

105. Johansson K, Nuutila L, Virtanen H, et al. Preoperative education for orthopaedic patients: systematic review. J Adv Nurs 2005;50:212–23.

106. McDonald S, Hetrick S, Green S. Pre-operative education for hip or knee replacement. Cochrane Database Syst Rev 2004;(5):CD003526.

107. Vila H Jr, Smith RA, Augustyniak MJ, et al. The efficacy and safety of pain management before and after implementation of hospital-wide pain management standards: is patient safety compromised by treatment based solely on numerical pain ratings? Anesth Analg 2005;101:474–80 table of contents.

108. Turk DC, Dworkin RH, Burke LB, et al. Developing patient-reported outcome measures for pain clinical trials: IMMPACT recommendations. Pain 2006;125:208–15.

109. Turk DC, Dworkin RH, McDermott MP, et al. Analyzing multiple endpoints in clinical trials of pain treatments: IMMPACT recommendations. Initiative on methods, measurement, and pain assessment in clinical trials. Pain 2008;139:485–93.

Preoperative Evaluation and Preparation of Patients for Orthopedic Surgery

Richard B. Abel, MD, Meg A. Rosenblatt, MD*

KEYWORDS

- Preoperative evaluation • Perioperative Surgical Home
- Orthopedic surgical patients

KEY POINTS

- The Perioperative Surgical Home model of patient care is a patient-centered, physician-led, multidisciplinary system of care for surgical patients that spans the entire surgical experience.
- Medical conditions that frequently require patients to undergo orthopedic procedures include ankylosing spondylitis, scoliosis, rheumatoid arthritis, and hemophilia.
- Each comorbidity has specific considerations for anesthesiologists during the preoperative evaluation.
- Blood conservation strategies should be considered and may be initiated during a preoperative evaluation.
- Preoperative teaching may increase patients' acceptance of regional anesthetic and analgesic techniques.

INTRODUCTION

Appropriate preoperative evaluation and preparation of patients for orthopedic surgery is an essential component of patient management. During the evaluation, a patient's preexisting medical comorbidities must be identified and explored. A detailed interview can occasionally reveal a patient history suggesting occult disease. For example, dyspnea on exertion first reported to an anesthesiologist may herald undiagnosed congestive heart failure, pulmonary hypertension, or ischemic heart disease. With a complete evaluation, the need for further diagnostic testing and medical management can more judiciously be prescribed. Along with a complete history,

Neither author has any relationship with a commercial company that has a financial interest in the subject matter or materials discussed in this article.
Department of Anesthesiology, The Icahn School of Medicine at Mount Sinai Medical Center, Box 1010, One Gustave L. Levy Place, New York, NY 10029, USA
* Corresponding author.
E-mail address: meg.rosenblatt@mountsinai.org

physical examination in orthopedic patients must be focused not only on the cardio-pulmonary system and the airway but must also include the neuromuscular system. The overall goals of the preanesthetic evaluation are shown in **Box 1**.

In 2011, the American Society of Anesthesiologists (ASA) formed the Committee on Future Models of Anesthesia Practice, in order to explore ways to provide quality patient care as well as reduce costs and improve efficiency. This group is currently developing the Perioperative Surgical Home (PSH). The goals of the PSH are multifaceted: to improve health care quality, enhance patient experience, increase anesthesiologist value, and streamline medical spending. The ASA's approach to the PSH calls for early patient engagement, decreased preoperative testing redundancy, improved operating room efficiency, and postsurgical care initiatives and planning; in essence to involve the anesthesiologist in every aspect of the surgical patients care.[1] In the ever-changing environment of clinical medicine it has become imperative for patients to be evaluated in a preoperative clinic before the day of surgery. Anesthesiologists often meet patients only minutes before entering the operating room and interact with them mainly through their postoperative visit, and this approach provides the anesthesiologist little time to adequately evaluate and manage patients. The PSH model attempts to remedy these shortcomings by creating "a patient-centered, physician-led system of coordinated care striving for better health care and reduced costs of care."[2]

RISK STRATIFICATION

One of the main goals of anesthesiologists is to evaluate patients for underlying cardiovascular disease in order to risk stratify patients and potentially alter management. Each year, thousands of patients have severe cardiovascular complications that contribute to increased perioperative morbidity and mortality.[3]

Originally developed in 1977 and updated in 1999 by Goldman and colleagues[4] as a tool to assist in stratifying patients with cardiovascular disease for noncardiac surgery, the Revised Cardiac Risk Index (RCRI) determined 6 predictors of cardiac morbidity and mortality. These predictors are shown in **Box 2**.[5] Not only does the RCRI allow for cardiovascular risk stratification, it provides anesthesiologists a screening tool to determine which patients might benefit from further diagnostic testing, medical therapy, or more invasive intraoperative monitoring. The American College of Cardiology and the American Heart Association (ACC/AHA) guidelines for preoperative testing for

---

Box 1
Goals and objectives of the preoperative evaluation of patients presenting for orthopedic surgery

Risk stratification

Anticipate and potentially prevent complications

Manage preoperative medications

Propose blood conservation strategies

Discussion of anesthetic plan

Perform preoperative education

Respond to patient questions

Plan for appropriate postoperative care

Box 2
Risk factors for major cardiac complication in patients undergoing noncardiac surgery

High-risk type of surgery

History of ischemic heart disease

History of congestive heart failure

History of cerebrovascular disease

Insulin-dependent diabetes

Preoperative serum creatinine greater than 2.0 mg/dL

Adapted from Lee TH, Marcantonio ER, Mangione CM, et al. Derivation and prospective validation of a simple index for prediction of cardiac risk of major noncardiac surgery. Circulation 1999;100:1045; with permission.

---

noncardiac surgery recently recommended noninvasive stress testing only for patients with active cardiac conditions or for patients with multiple cardiac risk factors who have poor functional status.[6] A few years after the ACC/AHA published their guidelines, a retrospective study on cardiac stress testing before major noncardiac surgery suggested that patients who underwent stress testing had reduced hospital mortality, lower 1-year mortality, and shorter hospital stays.[7]

Initiation of pharmacotherapy before certain surgeries may also decrease perioperative complications through risk modification. Although the Perioperative Ischemic Evaluation Study (POISE) highlights the caution physicians should exercise in universally initiating β-blocker therapy in surgical patients,[8] there is significant evidence that β-blockers play a role in decreasing cardiovascular complications in high-risk patients.[9] Statin therapy (agents that lower cholesterol levels by inhibiting 3-hydroxy-3-methyl-glutaryl-CoA [HMG-CoA] reductase) has also been highlighted as a means of modifying patient operative risks. Some experts recommend prescribing statin medications as early as possible before surgery, and perhaps continuing lifelong postoperatively.[10] Evaluation of patients before surgery also provides anesthesiologists with key information to anticipate the potential need for intraoperative vasoactive medical therapy or for invasive monitors such as transesophageal echocardiography, arterial blood pressure catheters, or central venous access.

Rather than relying on patient comorbidities and noninvasive testing to predict perioperative cardiac risk, the best guide to understanding patient cardiopulmonary status and prognosis remains exercise tolerance.[11] The metabolic equivalent of task (MET) has long been held as the gold standard by which to evaluate patient physical capacity. For example, a patient's ability to perform activities of daily living or climb 1 flight of stairs is roughly equivalent to 4 to 5 METs. Multiple studies have shown that a patient's ability to perform activities greater than 4 METs is associated with a decreased risk of perioperative cardiovascular events.[7]

PATIENTS WITH HIP (FEMUR) FRACTURES

Although risk stratification and preoperative optimization are important in the preoperative evaluation of orthopedic patients for elective procedures, one group of patients deserves special consideration. Operative delay may be associated with increased mortality in patients with hip fractures. A review of 16 prospective and retrospective observational studies assessed the timing of surgery and mortality in 257,367 patients.

A 48-hour delay from the time of admission was used to define an operative delay, and it was determined that the odds of 30-day mortality increased by 41% and 1 year all-cause mortality by 32% when surgery occurred with delay.[12] Using data from the National Patient Safety Agency, Panesar and colleagues[13] studied 4521 patients with hip fracture, and 96% of them experienced harm from delay of their repairs. They suggested that these patients be risk stratified according to their medical morbidities (hypovolemia, accelerated hypertension, untreated infection, symptomatic arrhythmia, cardiopulmonary dysfunction) and that clinicians should attempt to mitigate these conditions and then repair as soon as possible. For evaluating patients with proximal femoral fractures, there is evidence to support the early placement of fascia iliaca blocks for pain management to provide superior or equal pain relief compared with other forms of analgesia, while decreasing the deleterious side effects of systemic opioids.[14]

PREOPERATIVE TESTING

The traditional practice of having every patient undergo a full battery of preoperative testing is slowly giving way to limiting studies to the minimum amount needed to provide patient-focused and procedure-focused information. The National Physicians Alliance, through a foundation of the American Board of Internal Medicine (ABIM), undertook a project titled Promoting Good Stewardship in Clinical Practice, which identified 5 activities in family medicine, internal medicine, and pediatrics in which physicians in their respective specialties could alter their behaviors and ultimately produce an improvement in the quality of care delivered.[15] This notion has expanded to the ABIM's Choose Wisely campaign, which aims to promote dialogue between physicians and patients across many other specialties. The campaign helps patients choose necessary evidence-based care that limits potential harm. Two of the 5 activities that the ASA has identified specifically address preoperative medical procedures and testing that should be reviewed by anesthesiologists and patients alike. The first states that baseline laboratory studies (complete blood counts, metabolic panels, coagulation studies) in patients without significant systemic disease undergoing low-risk surgery should not be obtained when significant blood loss or fluid shifts are not expected. The second limits the need for baseline cardiac diagnostic testing in asymptomatic, stable patients with known cardiac disease undergoing low-risk or moderate-risk noncardiac surgery. The full list of ASA Choose Wisely initiatives can be found at http://www.choosingwisely.org/doctor-patient-lists/american-society-of-anesthesiologists/.

MEDICAL CONDITIONS THAT FREQUENTLY REQUIRE PATIENTS TO UNDERGO ORTHOPEDIC PROCEDURES
Ankylosing Spondylitis

Patients with ankylosing spondylitis (AS) commonly present for orthopedic surgery and pose numerous challenges necessitating preoperative evaluation and preparation by an anesthesiologist. AS is an autoimmune inflammatory disease that causes painful spondyloarthropathy primarily affecting the spine and sacroiliac joints. It typically presents in the second and third decades of life.[16] Prevalence of AS is approximately 1%, and many cases are associated with genetic inheritance of the human leukocyte antigen B27. As the disease progresses, AS involvement of the spine commonly leads to traumatic or spontaneous fractures, chronic pain, cervical instability, and severe kyphoscoliosis requiring therapeutic surgery.

The main preoperative anesthetic concerns for patients with AS are airway management and the cardiopulmonary manifestations of the disease. Atlanto-occipital subluxation is a possibility in patients with AS, which warrants preoperative plain radiographs to rule out the condition in patients with advanced disease. The temporomandibular joint is another site that is commonly involved, necessitating a thorough airway examination specifically to evaluate mouth opening and mandibular protrusion capabilities. As part of the airway management, many experts recommend performing an awake fiberoptic endotracheal intubation because of the frequent concurrent disease involvement of the cervical spine and temporomandibular joint.[17]

In severe cases of AS, patients can develop severe kyphoscoliosis causing a fixed thoracic deformity and leading to pulmonary implications. Pulmonary function tests (PFTs) often show a restrictive lung disease pattern with reduced total lung capacity. For reasons unknown, AS is also associated with an increased incidence of parenchymal lung disease leading to fibrosis and decreased diffusion capacity.[18] AS occasionally affects the heart by infiltrating the wall of the aorta, which can lead to aortic insufficiency.[19]

Scoliosis

Scoliosis is a lateral and rotational deformity of the axial spine that involves up to 5% of the American population. Although some cases can be linked to specific causes such as underlying neuromuscular diseases, most cases are idiopathic. Most patients with scoliosis never require surgical intervention. For patients with scoliosis who elect to undergo surgical intervention, the main goal of the procedure is to prevent the progression of disease rather than correction of existing deformity.[20]

Preoperative assessment should be focused on the pulmonary and cardiovascular systems, because they are the most prominently affected by the disease. Deformity of the thoracic spine can lead to development of restrictive lung disease, warranting preoperative PFTs to assess the extent of restriction and baseline vital capacity values. Obtaining oxygen tension levels, measured via arterial blood gas, may be justified in the presurgical setting because relative hypoxia often develops in patients with scoliosis with extensive lung involvement. Thoracic surgery for scoliosis often involves an anterior approach to the spine, necessitating one lung ventilation to allow for appropriate surgical exposure. The stress of intrathoracic surgery on the pulmonary system coupled with underlying lung disease places patients with scoliosis having thoracic spine surgery at an increased risk for requiring postoperative ventilator support.[21]

Without surgical intervention, many patients with severe scoliosis die by the age of 50 years from respiratory failure, pulmonary hypertension, or right heart failure.[22] Cardiovascular preoperative evaluation should be designed to determine patient functional capacity and extent of pulmonary hypertension and right heart failure. Patients with poor exercise tolerance may require more extensive preoperative diagnostic testing, such as transthoracic echocardiography to evaluate right ventricular systolic function or right heart catheterization to accurately determine pulmonary artery pressures.

Rheumatoid Arthritis

Approximately 1% of people carry the diagnosis of rheumatoid arthritis (RA), a progressive autoimmune disease that classically affects synovial joints. RA is a chronic disease with episodic inflammatory changes that occur in conjunction with progressive joint destruction and structural demise. Because of the disease's propensity to involve the musculoskeletal system, patients with RA frequently present for orthopedic procedures throughout the course of their lives.

Some of the joints that RA often affects that are of specific interest to the anesthesiologist include the atlantoaxial, temporomandibular, and the cricoarytenoid joints. Atlantoaxial subluxation is a serious concern in patients with RA, often causing neck pain, stiffness, radiculopathy, and sometimes quadriplegia or sudden death.[23,24] Patients with RA with nonspecific neck pain or stiffness should initially be evaluated with plain radiographs and often require further work-up for atlantoaxial joint disease using MRI before surgery. For patients presenting for cervical spine surgery or with a known history of atlantoaxial subluxation, care must be taken to limit neck manipulation during endotracheal intubation. Many experts suggest preinduction positioning of patients and performance of a fiberoptic intubation to limit cervical neck extension or flexion. Atlantoaxial disease is sometimes accompanied by temporomandibular joint involvement, further complicating airway management by limiting mouth opening because of either discomfort or joint destruction. There are also several case reports in which RA involving the cricoarytenoid joint led to upper airway obstruction and the need for an emergent surgical airway in the perioperative period.[25,26]

RA can manifest in numerous areas outside the musculoskeletal system. Patients are at an increased risk for coronary artery disease, atrial fibrillation, and heart failure.[27,28] Owing to its inflammatory disease process, patients with RA are prone to development of infiltrative myocarditis and pericarditis.[29] Pulmonary complications of RA include pleural disease, interstitial lung disease, and rheumatoid lung nodules. Many of the medications used to treat the disease can lead to drug-induced lung toxicity with a multitude of clinical manifestations.[30] Long-term RA antiinflammatory therapy with corticosteroids occasionally leads to diabetes and functional adrenal suppression.

Hemophilia

Hemophilia is a group of hereditary genetic disorders that cause bleeding diatheses. Factor VIII deficiency, known as hemophilia A, accounts for 80% of the hemophiliac population. The coagulopathy that develops from a lack of factor VIII places patients at high risk for intra-articular and intramuscular hemorrhage. Repetitive hemarthroses cause a chronic proliferative synovitis and cartilage destruction that leads to hemophilic arthropathy, whereas intramuscular bleeding can lead to contracture and atrophy of muscles.[31] Because of the propensity for bleeding to involve the musculoskeletal system, hemophiliacs frequently require orthopedic procedures that include contracture releases, arthroscopies, osteotomies, and joint arthroplasties.

In order to safely care for a patient with hemophilia, the anesthesiologist must be in close communication with the patient's hematologist and understand appropriate transfusion therapy to mitigate the potential for perioperative bleeding and hemorrhage. Since its advent, recombinant factor VIII (rFVIII) has been the mainstay for the prevention of bleeding and the treatment of active hemorrhage in these patients.[32] Anesthesiologists must consult with hematologists to discuss the individual patient's intrinsic levels of factor VIII, the presence of factor inhibitors that often occurs after initiation of rFVIII therapy, and the appropriate dose and timing of administration of rFVIII in the perisurgical period.

Adjuncts are often used in combination with rFVIII not only to work synergistically in preventing bleeding but also to decrease the amount of rFVIII needed, because of its high cost and limited availability. Desmopressin is a vasopressin analogue that increases factor VIII and von Willebrand factor plasma activity. Antifibrinolytics, like tranexamic acid and ε-aminocaproic acid, are lysine analogues that can be administered in conjunction with rFVIII and desmopressin to inhibit fibrinolysis. Because of the limited half-life of all the medications used in the management of hemophilia-related bleeding, patients undergoing invasive procedures should be observed postoperatively in a monitored setting.[33]

PERIOPERATIVE MEDICATION MANAGEMENT

Another role in which the PSH helps streamline patient care is in preoperative and postoperative pharmacotherapy management. Medication decisions in the preoperative period are often multifaceted, with specific concerns for chronic medical conditions, anesthetic implications, and surgical consequences. Although the list of potential preoperative medications is extensive, this article focuses on those that anesthesiologists most commonly encounter and those that may have the most substantial medical impact on patient care perioperatively.

For years, the wealth of evidence-based guidelines for perioperative medication management was lacking, forcing most decisions to be made empirically. Patients often presented on the day of surgery having refrained from taking any of their chronic medications. Although there is a lack of controlled randomized trials to tailor preoperative medication management, there are several expert recommendations and studies to serve as guides.

One of the most prevalent comorbidities in patients is essential hypertension, which is experienced by more than a quarter of the American population.[34] For the most part, antihypertensive medications should be continued in the perioperative setting with the exception of patients taking angiotensin-converting enzyme inhibitors (ACE-Is), angiotensin receptor blockers (ARBs), or diuretics. Patients on chronic ACE-Is and ARBs are at increased risk of significant hypotension during general anesthesia.[35] One study showed significant hemodynamic instability in patients chronically managed on a combination of ACE-Is/ARBs and diuretics.[36] Withholding ACE-Is/ARBs must be weighed against the potential for the patient to present with increased blood pressures on the day of surgery. Most experts recommend discontinuing diuretics in the perioperative period in an attempt to avoid hypovolemic hypotension.[37]

Antithrombotic therapy in the perioperative period has received much attention in recent years. For some time, patients were told to discontinue all antiplatelet medication more than a week before surgery, independent of the indication for the therapy. Stopping antithrombotic medications can have a significant impact on patient morbidity and mortality. Communication between anesthesiologist, surgeon, and prescribing physician as to the indication and necessity for antiplatelet therapy should be made when possible. Patients with recent percutaneous coronary interventions, especially stenting, are at increased risk of coronary thrombosis if antithrombotic medication is discontinued in the perioperative period. In addition to the hypercoagulable state that surgery induces, cessation of antithrombotic therapy can cause a rebound hypercoagulability, putting patients at an even higher risk of a thromboembolic event.[38] The risk of surgical hemorrhage must be weighed against that of a potentially catastrophic thrombotic event in patients with recent coronary stents. The ACC/AHA and the Society for Cardiovascular Angiography and Interventions currently recommend continued dual antiplatelet therapy with daily aspirin 325 mg and clopidogrel 75 mg, for a minimum of 1 month following bare metal stenting, 3 months after sirolimus drug-eluting stent (DES) placement, and 6 months following paclitaxel DES insertion.[39] The ACC/AHA recommends that patients should ideally be treated with dual antiplatelet therapy for at least 1 year after percutaneous cardiac interventions.[39] However, a recent retrospective cohort study of major adverse cardiac events in the perioperative period in patients with coronary stents suggests that patient risk factors and comorbidities may be better tools to guide the duration of antiplatelet therapy than time from stent placement.[40] At present, these investigators recommend continuing dual antiplatelet therapy during the perioperative period unless there is significant risk of hemorrhage or the patient is undergoing surgeries in which perioperative bleeding could result in significant morbidity, such as spinal canal, intracranial, or posterior eye surgery. If concomitant risk factors are absent and the hemorrhagic risk is significant, withdrawing thienopyridines while maintaining aspirin is a reasonable approach.[41]

BLOOD CONSERVATION STRATEGIES

Some orthopedic procedures portend a high risk for significant perioperative bleeding and the need for allogenic blood transfusion. For years, physicians have attempted to devise alternatives to allogenic blood transfusion, given the risks and complications that can be incurred. Adjuncts that have been offered to patients are preoperative iron, erythropoietin supplementation, and autologous blood donation. Erythropoietin acts by stimulating the patient's own bone marrow to increase production of red blood cells. A systematic review of randomized trials found that erythropoietin therapy was effective in decreasing the need for perioperative blood transfusion during orthopedic and cardiac surgery, but at the cost of increased thromboembolic events.[42] Autologous blood transfusion is another alternative that is often offered to surgical patients who want to limit exposure to allogeneic blood products. The 3 methods of autologous donation are preoperative blood donation, intraoperative blood salvage, and acute normovolemic hemodilution (ANH).[43] Preoperative blood donation requires patients to predonate their own blood at a donation bank. The predonated blood is then processed and stored for potential future autologous transfusion. Red blood cell salvage uses a salvage system to recoup blood lost in the surgical field and administer the washed red blood cells back to the patient. ANH, performed on the day of surgery, involves the collection of blood from the patient and replacement of that volume with crystalloid. The whole blood is returned to the patient toward the conclusion of the operation, once surgical hemostasis has been obtained. Although autologous blood transfusion may seem like a panacea to prevent allogenic blood transfusions, it has limitations. Autologous blood transfusion therapy is expensive (time to donate, storage costs), carries its own risks of infection and potential clerical errors, and is logistically difficult to accomplish. A recent retrospective study of total hip arthroplasty surgeries suggests that the use of preoperative autologous blood donation mainly benefits anemic patients,[44] but patients who predonate blood too close to the date of surgery may present to the operating room with a relative anemia and incur a greater risk for the need for transfusion than those patients who have not predonated blood. Allogenic blood transfusion still plays a major role in perioperative transfusion therapy but, as minimally invasive techniques of surgery are perfected, it is hoped that the need for transfusion and the role of techniques for preventing allogeneic transfusion will be minimized.

PATIENT EDUCATION

One of the major goals in the initiation of the PSH is to have anesthesiologists educate patients about the perioperative experience, which includes preoperative medication management, intraoperative anesthetic options, and plans for postoperative analgesia. The anesthesiologist can also attempt to alleviate the fear and anxiety that patients may have regarding the perioperative period. More than 50 years ago, Egbert and colleagues[45] discussed the psychological importance of the preoperative interaction and education of patients in providing anxiolysis to patients. Preoperative patient education also offers patients the tools to make educated decisions about their care and to be able to provide informed consent for anesthetic plans and procedures.

The advantages of regional anesthesia compared with general anesthesia in the intraoperative and postoperative periods for patients undergoing orthopedic surgery are numerous, and include providing postoperative analgesia, increased cardiovascular stability, avoidance of airway manipulation, potential for postanesthesia care unit bypass, lower incidence of postoperative nausea and vomiting, and greater patient satisfaction.[46,47] Introduction to neuraxial and single-shot or continuous catheter techniques should ideally occur before the day of surgery. In this way, fears about discomfort during the performance of the block and about being awake during surgery can be allayed, and therapeutic benefits of having analgesia that extends into the postoperative period can be explained.

FUTURE CONSIDERATIONS AND SUMMARY

Anesthesiologists traditionally meet their patients only before entering the surgical theater. With a preoperative evaluation clinic, which is essential to the PSH model, patients should present to the operating room medically optimized and well informed about their anesthetic plans and their respective risks or benefits.[48,49] The preoperative evaluation of orthopedic surgical patients should ideally minimize risks, medications should appropriately be managed, blood conservation strategies initiated, plans for anesthesia and postoperative analgesia known, and patient anxiety alleviated. The PSH should ensure the active participation of anesthesiologists in all aspects of patient care.

REFERENCES

1. Schweitzer M, Fahy B, Leib M, et al. The perioperative surgical home model. American Society of Anesthesiologists Newsletter 2012;118:58–9.
2. Available at: https://www.asahq.org/For-Members/Perioperative-Surgical-Home. aspx. Accessed March 1, 2014.
3. Devereaux PJ, Goldman L, Cook DJ, et al. Perioperative cardiac events in patients undergoing noncardiac surgery: a review of the magnitude of the problem, the pathophysiology of the events and methods to estimate and communicate risk. CMAJ 2005;173:627–34.
4. Goldman L, Caldera DL, Nussbaum SR, et al. Multifactorial index of cardiac risk in noncardiac surgical procedures. N Engl J Med 1977;297:845.
5. Lee TH, Marcantonio ER, Mangione CM, et al. Derivation and prospective validation of a simple index for prediction of cardiac risk of major noncardiac surgery. Circulation 1999;100:1043–9.
6. Fleisher LA, Beckman JA, Brown KA. ACC/AHA 2007 guidelines on perioperative cardiovascular evaluation and care for noncardiac surgery: a report of the American College of Cardiology/American Heart Association Task Force on Practice Guidelines (Writing Committee to revise the 2002 Guidelines on Perioperative Cardiovascular Evaluation for Non-Cardiac Surgery). J Am Coll Cardiol 2007; 50:e159–241.
7. Wijeysundera D, Beattle W, Elliot R, et al. Non-invasive cardiac stress testing before elective major non-cardiac surgery: population based cohort study. BMJ 2010;340:b5526.
8. POISE Study Group. Effects of extended-release metoprolol succinate in patients undergoing non-cardiac surgery (POISE trial): a randomised controlled trial. Lancet 2008;371:1839–47.

9. Fleisher LA, Beckman JA, Brown KA, et al. ACC/AHA 2006 guideline update on perioperative cardiovascular evaluation for noncardiac surgery: focused update on perioperative beta-blocker therapy: a report of the American College of Cardiology/American Heart Association Task Force on Practice Guidelines (Writing Committee to Update the 2002 Guidelines on Perioperative Cardiovascular Evaluation for Noncardiac Surgery). Circulation 2006;113:2662–74.

10. Biccard BM, Sear JW, Foëx P. Statin therapy: a potentially useful peri-operative intervention in patients with cardiovascular disease. Anaesthesia 2005;60: 1106–14.

11. Reilly DF, McNeely MJ, Doerner D, et al. Self-reported exercise tolerance and the risk of serious perioperative complications. Arch Intern Med 1999;159:2185–92.

12. Shiga T, Wajima Z, Ohe Y. Is operative delay associated with increased mortality of hip fracture patients? Systemic review, meta-analysis, and meta regression. Can J Anaesth 2008;55:135–9.

13. Panesar SS, Simunovic N, Bhandari M. When should we operate on elderly patients with a hip fracture? It's about time! Surgeon 2012;10:185–8.

14. Chesters A, Atkinson P. Fascia iliaca block for pain relief from proximal femoral fracture in the emergency department: a review of the literature. Emerg Med J 2014. http://dx.doi.org/10.1136/emermed-2013-203073.

15. Good Stewardship Working Group. "Top 5" lists in primary care: meeting the responsibility of professionalism. Arch Intern Med 2011;171:1385–90.

16. Akkoc N, Khan MA. Epidemiology of ankylosing spondylitis and related spondyloarthropathies. In: Weisman MH, Reveille JD, van der Heijde D, editors. Ankylosing spondylitis and the spondyloarthropathies. London: Mosby; 2005. p. 117–31.

17. Woodward LJ, Kam PC. Ankylosing spondylitis: recent developments and anesthetic implications. Anaesthesia 2009;64:540–8.

18. Berdal G, Halvorsen S, van der Heijde D, et al. Restrictive pulmonary function is more prevalent in patients with ankylosing spondylitis than in matched population controls and is associated with impaired spinal mobility: a comparative study. Arthritis Res Ther 2012;14:R19.

19. Slobodin G, Naschitz JE, Zuckerman E, et al. Aortic involvement in rheumatic diseases. Clin Exp Rheumatol 2006;24(2 Suppl 41):S41–7.

20. Peterson LE, Nachemson AL. Prediction of progression of the curve in girls who have adolescent idiopathic scoliosis of moderate severity. J Bone Joint Surg Am 1995;77:823–7.

21. McDonnelll MF, Glassman SD, Dimar JR, et al. Perioperative complications of anterior procedures of the spine. J Bone Joint Surg Am 1996;16:293–303.

22. Pehrsson K, Larsson S, Oden A, et al. Long-term follow-up of patients with untreated scoliosis. A study of mortality, causes of death, and symptoms. Spine (Phila PA 1976) 1992;17:1091–6.

23. Bollensen E, Schonle PW, Braun U, et al. An unnoticed dislocation of the dens axis in a patient with primary chronic polyarthritis undergoing intensive therapy. Anaesthesist 1991;40:294–7.

24. Takenaka I, Urakami Y, Aoyama K, et al. Severe subluxation in the sniffing position in a rheumatoid patient with anterior atlantoaxial subluxation. Anesthesiology 2004;101:1235–7.

25. Kolman J, Morris I. Cricoarytenoid arthritis: a cause of acute upper airway obstruction in rheumatoid arthritis. Can J Anesth 2002;49:729–32.

26. Chen JJ, Branstetter BF, Myers EN. Cricoarytenoid rheumatoid arthritis: an important consideration in aggressive lesions of the larynx. AJNR Am J Neuroradiol 2005;26:970–2.

27. Gabriel SE. Heart disease and rheumatoid arthritis: understanding the risks. Ann Rheum Dis 2010;69(Suppl 1):i61–4.
28. Lindhardsen J, Ahlehoff O, Gislason GH, et al. Risk of atrial fibrillation and stroke in rheumatoid arthritis: Danish nationwide cohort study. BMJ 2012;344: e1257.
29. Guedes C, Bianchi-Fior P, Cormier B, et al. Cardiac manifestations of rheumatoid arthritis: a case control transesophageal echocardiography study in 30 patients. Arthritis Rheum 2001;45:129–35.
30. Libby D, White DA. Pulmonary toxicity of drugs used to treat systemic autoimmune diseases. Clin Chest Med 1998;19:809–21.
31. Raffini L, Manno C. Modern management of haemophilic arthropathy. Br J Haematol 2007;136:777–87.
32. Manco-Johnson MJ, Abshire TC, Shapiro AD, et al. Prophylaxis versus episodic treatment to prevent joint disease in boys with severe hemophilia. N Engl J Med 2007;357:535–44.
33. Srivastava A, Brewer AK, Mauser-Bunschoten EP, et al, Treatment Guidelines Working Group of the World Federation of Hemophilia. Guidelines for the management of hemophilia. Haemophilia 2013;19:e1–47.
34. Burt V, Whelton P, Brown C, et al. Prevalence of hypertension in the US adult population. Results from the Third National Health and Nutrition Examination Survey, 1988-1991. Hypertension 1995;25:305–13.
35. Lee YK, Na SW, Kwak YL, et al. Effect of pre-operative angiotensin-converting enzyme inhibitors on haemodynamic parameters and vasoconstrictor requirements in patients undergoing off-pump coronary artery bypass surgery. J Int Med Res 2005;33:693–702.
36. Kheterpal S, Khondaparast O, Shanks A, et al. Chronic angiotensin-converting enzyme inhibitor or angiotensin receptor blocker therapy combined with diuretic therapy is associated with increased episodes of hypotension in non-cardiac surgery. J Cardiothorac Vasc Anesth 2008;22:180–6.
37. Christopher W. Perioperative medication management: general principles and practical applications. Cleve Clin J Med 2009;76(Suppl 4):S126–32.
38. Genewain U, Haeberli A, Straub PW, et al. Rebound after cessation of oral anticoagulant therapy: the biochemical evidence. Br J Haematol 1996;92:479–85.
39. Smith SC Jr, Feldman TE, Hirshfeld JW Jr, et al. ACC/AHA/SCAI 2005 guideline update for percutaneous coronary intervention: a report of the American College of Cardiology/American Heart Association Task Force of Practice Guidelines (ACC/AHA/SCAI Writing Committee to Update the 2001 Guidelines for Percutaneous Coronary Intervention). J Am Coll Cardiol 2006;47:216–35.
40. Hawn MT, Graham LA, Richman JS, et al. Risk of major adverse cardiac events following noncardiac surgery in patients with coronary stents. JAMA 2013;310: 1462–72.
41. Eisenberg MJ, Richard PR, Libersan D, et al. Safety of short-term discontinuation of antiplatelet therapy in patients with drug-eluting stents. Circulation 2009;119: 1634–42.
42. Laupacis A, Fergusson D. Erythropoietin to minimize perioperative blood transfusion: a systemic review of randomized trials. The International Study of Perioperative Transfusion (ISPOT) Investigators. Transfus Med 1998;8:309–17.
43. Walunj A, Babb A, Sharpe R. Autologous blood transfusion. CEACCP 2006;6:192–6. Available at: http://ceaccp.oxfordjournals.org/content/6/5/192.full.
44. Boettner F, Altneu E, Sculco T. Nonanemic patients do not benefit from autologous blood donation before total hip replacement. HSS J 2010;6:66–70.

45. Egbert LD, Gattit G, Turndorf H, et al. The value of the preoperative visit by an anesthetist. A study of doctor-patient rapport. JAMA 1963;185:553–5.
46. O'Donnell B, Iohom G. Regional anesthesia techniques for ambulatory orthopedic surgery. Curr Opin Anaesthesiol 2008;21:723–8.
47. Tetzlaff JE, Yoon HJ, Brems J. Patient acceptance of interscalene block for shoulder surgery. Reg Anesth 1993;18(1):30–3.
48. Kitts JB. The preoperative assessment: who is responsible? Can J Anaesth 1997; 44:1232–6.
49. Conway JB, Goldberg J, Chung F. Preadmission anesthesia consultation clinic. Can J Anaesth 1992;39:1051–7.

Setting Up an Acute Pain Management Service

Eric S. Schwenk, MD[a,*], Jaime L. Baratta, MD[a], Kishor Gandhi, MD, MPH, CPE[b], Eugene R. Viscusi, MD[a]

KEYWORDS

- Acute pain service • Multimodal analgesia • Continuous peripheral nerve block
- Epidural analgesia

KEY POINTS

- Specific, defined roles for acute pain management service (APMS) team members and the use of protocols can help improve patient care and eliminate uncertainty that could lead to errors.
- Opioid-tolerant patients comprise a large portion of APMS patients, and a thorough understanding of their needs, in addition to an emphasis on a multimodal approach, can lead to optimal outcomes.
- APMS attending physicians must stay current with new drugs and regional techniques so that the service can meet the needs of the increasingly complex patients and surgeries.

INTRODUCTION

An organized and integrated acute pain management service (APMS) is a requirement for delivery of high-quality pain management in an increasingly complex health care environment driven by patient satisfaction. Aggressive techniques for acute pain management require an attentive, well-trained, and dedicated staff of physicians, nurses, and pharmacists, all with a consistent set of goals: to provide safe, timely, and effective management of all acute pain scenarios. Current complex techniques require frequent surveillance and adjustment to assure consistent efficacy, quick adjustment for side effects, and care to avoid medication-related or technology-related errors. An organized approach to acute pain management with standardization of procedures, orders, and monitoring, along with an integrated interdisciplinary emphasis, is warranted.

Disclosures: E.S. Schwenk, J.L. Baratta, K. Gandhi have no financial disclosures. Research grants to my institution – AcelRx, Cumberland, Pacira; Consulting/honoraria – AcelRx, Cadence/Malinckrodt, Cubist, Salix, Pacira (E.R. Viscusi).
[a] Department of Anesthesiology, Thomas Jefferson University, Suite 8130, Gibbon Building, 111 South 11th Street, Philadelphia, PA 19107, USA; [b] Department of Anesthesiology, University Medical Center of Princeton, 1 Plainsboro Road, Plainsboro Township, NJ 08540, USA
* Corresponding author.
E-mail address: Eric.Schwenk@jefferson.edu

Anesthesiology Clin 32 (2014) 893–910
http://dx.doi.org/10.1016/j.anclin.2014.08.008
1932-2275/14/$ – see front matter © 2014 Elsevier Inc. All rights reserved.

anesthesiology.theclinics.com

MULTIMODAL APPROACH TO PAIN MANAGEMENT

One of the keys to developing and maintaining a successful APMS is the implementation of multimodal analgesia, which is the use of several pharmacologic agents with different mechanisms of action to treat pain. The goal is to minimize the side effects of each individual agent and target multiple pain receptors to provide optimum analgesia and facilitate recovery. In particular, minimizing opioids by making nonopioid agents the first-line treatment for pain should be emphasized whenever possible. Multimodal approaches, combined with accelerated recovery protocols, can reduce the length of stay in hospital.[1] Use of these protocols has become routine at the authors' institution; unless contraindicated, almost all patients typically receive acetaminophen (intravenous or oral form), a nonsteroidal anti-inflammatory drug (NSAID), a gabapentinoid (gabapentin or pregabalin), and an opioid, either via patient-controlled analgesia (PCA) or orally. Multimodal analgesia using an NSAID combined with an opioid is more effective than using opioids alone.[2] Similarly, the addition of gabapentin[3] or pregabalin[4] to a multimodal regimen can decrease opioid consumption and their related side effects.

When appropriate for the type of pain and surgery, local anesthetics are an excellent class of medication to incorporate, whether through a continuous peripheral nerve block (CPNB), continuous epidural infusion, or even intravenously. Local anesthetics are discussed elsewhere in this article.

Ketamine is a useful adjunct to a multimodal regimen, especially in opioid-tolerant patients or in those with neuropathic pain. Ketamine is an N-methyl-D-aspartate (NMDA)-receptor antagonist and potent analgesic. However, because it is a phencyclidine derivative, patients must be monitored for psychotropic side effects. Such surveillance typically involves frequent assessments by the APMS nurses. A protocol should be in place that prevents the use of ketamine by anyone outside of the APMS, especially in light of its potential for abuse. At the authors' institution, ketamine has been used with increasing frequency as a sedative in mechanically ventilated patients because of its lack of respiratory and cardiovascular depressive effects, and in patients with intractable migraine headaches, in whom there is emerging evidence that it may reduce the severity of the aura.[5] To summarize recommendations for ketamine use:

- Ketamine use should be restricted to the APMS.
- Patients receiving ketamine for analgesia should be monitored frequently for psychotropic side effects (hallucinations, dissociative sensation) and nystagmus.
- If the APMS is following a patient receiving ketamine, no special monitoring (eg, telemetry) is required.
- Although the acute pain nurse may be permitted to titrate the ketamine infusion rate, bolus doses should be given by a physician, such as the APMS resident.

STRUCTURE AND INDIVIDUAL ROLES WITHIN AN ACUTE PAIN MANAGEMENT SERVICE

An APMS consists of a team of providers who work together in distinct roles to care for patients in the perioperative period, and others having acute exacerbations of pain (eg, trauma, cancer, sickle cell crisis). The APMS is led by the director, who should be an anesthesiologist trained and experienced in the management of complex pain syndromes and in the performance of commonly requested regional anesthesia procedures, including thoracic epidurals, femoral nerve blocks (and, more recently, adductor canal blocks), and various brachial plexus blocks. This person's responsibilities include:

- Determining the direction of the service; defining the research, clinical, and educational goals of the service

- Developing policies and protocols for pain assessment and treatment
- Communicating with hospital administration and referring physicians
- Periodically reviewing quality indicators

The director can offer advice regarding the scope of the APMS and the appropriateness of referrals, and can attempt to resolve complicated questions regarding procedures and therapies. Cooperation with other specialties in a multidisciplinary team is often required, such as working with a palliative care specialist for patients with terminal cancer or consulting with a hematologist throughout the care of an opioid-tolerant patient with sickle cell disease. The director's role, and that of the other members of the APMS team, is summarized in **Table 1**.

The APMS attending staff includes other anesthesiologists experienced in pain management and regional anesthesia techniques. Whether this person rotates daily or on a weekly basis will vary depending on the institution and staff. He or she will lead rounds each day, and supervise any interventional procedures to be performed.

Table 1
Description of roles of members of an acute pain management service

Role	Description
Director	Determines direction of service Defines and coordinates clinical, educational, and research goals Develops pain policies and protocols Communicates with hospital administration, nursing management, referring physicians, and specialists Evaluates performance of all members of the team Periodically performs quality assurance
APMS attending	Leads daily patient rounds Performs and supervises regional anesthesia procedures Performs and supervises pain consultations Participates in educational and research goals and communicates any problems or issues with the director
APMS fellow/ resident	Participates in daily rounds Responds to acute pain consultation requests Performs regional anesthesia procedures (epidurals, peripheral nerve blocks) under supervision Answers pages and questions about routine pain management; refers complicated questions to the APMS attending Supervises interns and medical students performing consultations Participates in educational and research goals
Clinical nurse specialist	Coordinates services and provides continuity of care for patients Designs and implements educational programs for the department of nursing and patients Collects data and participates in quality assurance Assists the APMS director in development of goals, policies, protocols, and standards
APMS nurse	Keeps service pager and responds to calls about pain issues Frequently assesses the pain and medication side effects of patients on the APMS Using treatment protocols, adjusts pain medication regimen and frequently assesses efficacy of changes Provides reassurance to patients and nonpharmacologic therapies, including relaxation and distraction techniques

Abbreviation: APMS, acute pain management service.

The APMS fellow or resident will typically rotate through the service from a few days to a month at a time. Ideally he or she should remain on service for at least a week at a time to allow for continuity of care. It is the authors' experience that spending sporadic days on APMS benefits neither the fellow/resident nor the service, and can lead to omission of important information and confusion on the part of the trainee. In particular, junior residents can be especially prone to error during handoffs, which has also been demonstrated in the literature.[6] Continuity and communication is key to a well-organized APMS. Typical duties of the APMS fellow or resident and others are described in **Table 1**.

ROLE OF ACUTE PAIN MANAGEMENT SERVICE NURSES AND THE USE OF PROTOCOLS

At the authors' institution, there is an APMS nurse available by pager 24 hours a day, except for portions of the weekends, which are covered by residents. Although this structure may not be practical or possible at some institutions, it does allow for round-the-clock management of pain. In particular, the APMS nurse working overnight during the week can field routine pages and calls and recommend simple changes to a patient's regimen that are based on defined protocols and are within their scope of practice. For example, patients with CPNBs may need boluses of local anesthetic periodically, and at the authors' institution APMS nurses are permitted to give boluses of dilute local anesthetic via the infusion pump. Another example of an advantage of 24-hour APMS nurses is responding to calls about medication side effects. Often the patient's primary team is not familiar with dosing or side effects of pain medications, and APMS nurses can refer to written protocols and suggest treatment, such as antiemetics or antihistamines, for opioid-related side effects. In settings where round-the-clock dedicated pain nurses are not possible, it is critical to have dedicated and specially trained providers who proactively manage patients on the service.

An example of a nurse-driven protocol for the APMS is shown in **Fig. 1**. The clinical nurse specialist, in conjunction with the APMS director, can help develop protocols for various clinical scenarios, including the treatment of medication side effects, dosing of epidural or peripheral nerve catheters, and responding to calls from ambulatory patients who were discharged with a CPNB, among others. Although nurse practitioners have an advanced scope of practice and are able to enter orders themselves, the authors' experience with an APMS incorporating specially trained nurses with physician backup and well-crafted protocols and pathways within a set of pain management orders has shown this model to be effective.

INTRAVENOUS PATIENT-CONTROLLED ANALGESIA

Intravenous PCA involves patients self-administering small doses of opioid at predetermined intervals (lockout) to maintain analgesia. PCA provides superior analgesia and increased patient satisfaction in comparison with traditional, intermittent opioid bolus dosing.[7] PCA pumps can be programmed to deliver intermittent boluses on demand, either alone or with a basal infusion. Basal infusions should be reserved for opioid-tolerant patients because they can increase the risk of respiratory depression without improving analgesia.[8] Functions that can be programmed in a PCA pump include the demand dose, lockout time, total hourly dose, and basal infusion rate. An important point is that PCA is designed to maintain analgesia, not initiate it. Consequently, a loading dose of opioid is needed before starting a PCA pump to establish satisfactory analgesia.[9] It also follows from this that interruptions, whether caused by technical pump issues or disconnections from the pump for other reasons, will decrease the efficacy of PCA. Commonly used opioids in PCA pumps are listed in **Table 2**.

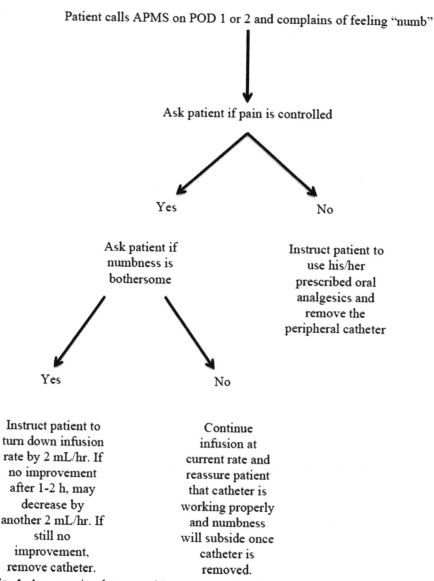

Patient calls APMS on POD 1 or 2 and complains of feeling "numb"

Ask patient if pain is controlled

Yes

No

Ask patient if numbness is bothersome

Instruct patient to use his/her prescribed oral analgesics and remove the peripheral catheter

Yes

No

Instruct patient to turn down infusion rate by 2 mL/hr. If no improvement after 1-2 h, may decrease by another 2 mL/hr. If still no improvement, remove catheter.

Continue infusion at current rate and reassure patient that catheter is working properly and numbness will subside once catheter is removed.

Fig. 1. An example of a nurse-driven protocol for the acute pain management service (APMS). POD, postoperative day.

Because the most common PCA-related problem is operator error,[10] maintaining consistency in drug concentration and pump settings is an important component of safe PCA management. Whenever possible, standard (equipotent) concentrations of opioids should be used (see **Table 2**). Modifications may need to be made for opioid-tolerant patients, but for the opioid-naïve, simple and standard is usually better. Verification of PCA pump programming by a second nurse can help reduce errors, as can the use of standard order entry forms. Suggestions for safe PCA use are given in **Box 1**. Protocols can help with the management of opioid-related side effects.

Table 2
Commonly used equianalgesic opioids for intravenous PCA

Opioid	Concentration (mg/mL)	Volume per Bolus (mL)	Lockout Interval (min)	Maximum Hourly Dose (mL)
Morphine	1	1–2	6	10–20
Hydromorphone	0.2	0.5–2	6–8	8–10
Fentanyl	0.01–0.02	1–2	6	10–20

Abbreviation: PCA, patient-controlled analgesia.

A simple but sometimes overlooked aspect of effective PCA is patient selection and comprehension. Although most adult patients can understand the principle of PCA, some cannot. Patients must be able to understand the need to self-administer doses and that no medication will be administered in the absence of patient effort. Obviously, patients whose tracheas are intubated and are receiving sedation cannot use PCA effectively. Patients at the extremes of age or those with dementia are poor PCA candidates.

Smart pump technology is advocated to reduce medication errors and programming errors. Although these newer pumps may help, errors continue to occur even with 2 nurses confirming drugs and programming. Therefore, careful organization, standardization, and expertise are mandated when PCA is used.

OPIOID-TOLERANT PATIENTS
Chronic Opioid Users

In a 2001 survey, 2% of all households reported taking an opioid for a month or longer[11]; meanwhile, opioid prescriptions have been rising steadily since 2001.[12] Many physicians treat opioid-tolerant patients, including those chronically taking opioids for pain, active opioid abusers, and those being treated for addiction with opioid agonists, on a daily basis in the hospital. On the APMS, opioid-tolerant patients commonly comprise at least half to two-thirds of the total number, and very often the percentage is greater. To effectively treat these patients a plan must be in place, beginning in the preoperative period or, ideally, during the surgical consultation or preoperative anesthesia evaluation. Patients taking opioids for chronic pain should be instructed to take their normal dose on the day of surgery.

As soon as possible, the opioid requirements of opioid-tolerant patients should be estimated based on the amount taken at home. An increase in opioid requirements

Box 1
Suggestions for safe use of patient-controlled analgesia (PCA)

- Use standard, equipotent PCA solutions
- Create protocols for respiratory depression monitoring, including the use of opioid antagonists
- Minimize errors through the use of standard order entry forms or electronic order entry systems
- Include supplemental nursing opioid boluses and medications for treatment of side effects as part of standard PCA orders
- Have 2 nurses verify PCA pump programming
- Reserve basal opioid infusions for opioid-tolerant patients; consider monitored settings

would be expected after surgery, but a strong emphasis on a multimodal approach, particularly incorporating ketamine and local anesthetic techniques, can minimize this increase. More potent opioids, such as hydromorphone and sufentanil, will be more effective than less potent ones, such as morphine. PCA self-administered doses need to be greater than for opioid-naïve patients, and for the highly tolerant patient a basal PCA infusion may be considered (a monitored setting with pulse oximetry and capnography is encouraged).

Although much effort and time will be focused on the management of opioids, the use of nonopioid agents should be emphasized. Regional anesthesia techniques using local anesthetics are ideal for decreasing opioid requirements. The APMS attending, in conjunction with regional anesthesiologists, can offer a variety of procedures to improve analgesia and decrease opioid consumption. In addition to the traditional surgeries, the APMS at the authors' institution has placed thoracic epidurals for trauma patients who have sustained rib fractures, and brachial plexus continuous blocks in patients with metastatic cancer affecting the shoulder and arm. The authors also routinely use low-dose subanesthetic infusions of ketamine in their opioid-tolerant population. Ketamine, an NMDA-receptor antagonist, is particularly useful for the treatment of neuropathic pain.[13] It also causes minimal effects on the cardiovascular and respiratory systems. Although less likely than with anesthetic doses, low-dose ketamine infusions may still cause dissociative side effects, so patients must be monitored frequently. Both APMS nurses and general floor nurses should be educated about the side effects for which to monitor, including hallucinations and vivid dreams. Nystagmus is fairly common and does not bother most patients, and is a benign side effect that should not limit therapy. Some patients may report vivid dreams but again are not typically bothered by them. Other multimodal agents, including NSAIDs, acetaminophen, gabapentinoids, and local anesthetics, should be maximized whenever possible. A summary of suggestions to manage opioid-tolerant patients is presented in **Box 2**.

Patients with Opioid Abuse or Addiction

With ever-increasing frequency, patients taking methadone for opioid abuse or addiction history are presenting for surgery. Although for the chronic opioid user a 2- to 3-fold increase in opioid requirements may be anticipated, advances in regional analgesia techniques and multimodal therapy have made this increase less common and

---

Box 2
Tips to successfully manage opioid-tolerant patients

- Define opioid requirements based on home doses
- Appreciate the 2- to 3-fold increase in opioid requirements that frequently occurs after surgery
- Continue extended-release and long-acting opioids on the day of surgery and resume them postoperatively as soon as feasible
- Choose more potent opioids, such as hydromorphone and sufentanil, rather than less potent opioids, such as morphine
- Maximize the use of nonopioid agents, especially local anesthetics (neuraxial blockade, peripheral nerve blockade, infiltration)
- When converting intravenous to oral opioids, consider overlapping PCA and oral medications for part of a day to monitor for efficacy of the chosen oral dose and make adjustments

less desirable. Patients taking methadone for opioid abuse or addiction should, if possible, receive their regular dose before surgery (which requires verification with the methadone clinic or authorized physician). Whenever the procedure is amenable, regional anesthesia techniques should be attempted to minimize the use of opioids and decrease the total amount of opioid given. Patients should be monitored postoperatively for respiratory depression because of the long half-life of methadone, especially if additional opioids are given. Methadone maintenance doses should generally be continued perioperatively.

Perhaps an even more challenging patient is the recovering opioid addict taking buprenorphine-naloxone (Suboxone), which is a combination of a μ-opioid receptor partial agonist (buprenorphine) and antagonist (naloxone). Because buprenorphine dissociates very slowly from μ-opioid receptors,[14] its clinical effects may persist beyond the time it is discontinued, and anesthesiologists are left with a difficult decision: continue the drug throughout the perioperative period or stop it. Ideally these patients should be evaluated and managed a week or more before surgery. If the decision is made to stop the medication for the perioperative period and use opioid-based analgesia, one must understand that high doses may be required, and some patients may be already experiencing hyperalgesia from abusing opioids.[15] However, buprenorphine itself may provide better analgesia than expected in patients who have been chronically taking opioids, possibly because of decreased hyperalgesia.[15] There is an emerging trend to continue buprenorphine perioperatively with modest dose adjustment as needed rather than convert to other opioids, particularly for less painful procedures. For pain that is more than mild, additional analgesics will likely be needed. The drug may then be restarted once the acute pain has subsided.

If the decision is made to continue buprenorphine-naloxone throughout the perioperative period, providers must understand that traditional opioid agonists will have limited efficacy. Regional anesthesia techniques and nonopioid agents should be applied whenever possible. If the expected pain level is mild, buprenorphine may provide adequate analgesia. For most procedures, additional analgesia may be required. Ketamine may be an effective alternative to opioids in this situation, and buprenorphine will not affect its efficacy.[16]

Often patients who have not been seen in a preoperative clinic will arrive for surgery and will have continued their buprenorphine-naloxone up until that time. For these patients discontinuation is not an option, so one is left to make the best of a less than ideal situation. Agents such as ketamine, acetaminophen, and NSAIDs, along with the use of regional techniques as indicated, can optimize the analgesia for these challenging patients.

NEURAXIAL ANALGESIA

Surgical procedures of the thorax, abdomen, and lower extremity are amenable to epidural analgesia for postoperative pain control. Epidural infusions have been proved to provide superior pain control when compared with intravenous opioids for thoracic and abdominal surgeries,[17] regardless of the choice of local anesthetic or addition of opioid.[18] Epidural analgesia also improves health-related outcomes, including fewer pulmonary complications (atelectasis, pulmonary infection, tracheal intubations), decreased postoperative ileus, and reduced 30-day mortality in intermediate- to high-risk noncardiac surgical patients.[19–21]

Neuraxial regional anesthesia techniques are not without risk, including postoperative backache, postdural puncture headache, local anesthetic systemic toxicity, total spinal anesthesia, neurologic injury, and spinal/epidural hematoma. The most dreaded complication is that of neurologic dysfunction secondary to spinal/epidural hematoma. Although the precise incidence is unknown, one article estimated an incidence of less than 1 in 150,000 epidural and less than 1 in 220,000 spinal anesthetics.[22] Studies show that the risk of clinically significant bleeding increases with age, abnormalities of the spine, the presence of an underlying coagulopathy, traumatic needle placement, and maintaining an indwelling neuraxial catheter during sustained anticoagulation.[22] APMS team members can play an important role in preventing spinal hematoma by staying current with their knowledge of old and new anticoagulants (**Tables 3** and **4**). This knowledge will help in lowering the chance of unintended catheter insertion or removal in an anticoagulated patient.

Optimal clinical application of epidural analgesia involves an APMS that is able to place epidural catheters before the patient reaches the operating theater. The APMS is typically notified with a specific need for an epidural placement before the patient reaches the holding area. Once the patient has been evaluated by the primary anesthesia provider, and proper consent (explanation of risks and benefits) and vascular access are obtained, the APMS team can place an epidural catheter in a safe, sterile, and efficient manner.

The choice of local anesthetic solution with or without additives and opioids varies by institution. The addition of epinephrine prolongs epidural blockade of both local anesthetics and opioids by inducing vasoconstriction in the epidural space and decreasing systemic absorption.[23] The addition of clonidine to a local anesthetic-opioid epidural mixture has also been shown to improve pain control after total knee arthroplasty, but with a decrease in blood pressure and heart rate.[24] Hypotension limits its utility. Ketamine, morphine, and epinephrine added to a ropivacaine infusion of patient-controlled epidural analgesia provided patients with better pain relief, suggesting an additive effect.[25]

The utility of adding opioids to the local anesthetic mixture is controversial. The combination of opioids and local anesthetic provides better dynamic pain control; however, adverse events may increase without vigilant monitoring.[26-29] Epidural opioids will diffuse into the surrounding tissue and cerebrospinal fluid.[30] Opioids bind to presynaptic and postsynaptic receptors in the dorsal horn of the spinal cord, and act to modulate nociceptive input from the periphery. The degree of opioid absorption in the tissue is determined by the lipophilicity of the drugs. Highly lipophilic drugs such as fentanyl and sufentanil preferentially get absorbed into adipose tissue, and minimal amounts enter the cerebrospinal fluid. Fentanyl and sufentanil are quickly absorbed by endothelial capillary membranes, and behave similarly to their intravenous formulations by binding to supraspinal (brainstem) opioid receptors. Drugs such as morphine and hydromorphone are hydrophilic and have greater bioavailability for opioid receptors in the spine. These agents have longer durations of action with higher side-effect profiles. Although epidural opioids added to local anesthetics may improve analgesia (but with increased side effects), it is not clear that they offer better analgesia when compared with opioid coadministration via another route. As with PCA, basal opioid infusions are linked to more respiratory depression. Hence, current guidelines recommend that all opioids be on demand and adjunctive to nonopioid analgesics.

Overall, the addition of opioids to local anesthetics in the epidural space can improve postoperative pain control. One of the key roles of the APMS in epidural management is monitoring for side effects. The risk of respiratory depression, which is manifested by a decreased respiratory rate and hypoxia, necessitates pulse oximetry monitoring postoperatively. An opioid antagonist, such as naloxone, should be part of standard PCA order sets, and all APMS team members should know and understand the treatment of respiratory depression and be familiar with the pharmacology of

Table 3
ASRA guidelines for neuraxial anesthesia with heparin, LMWH, and warfarin

Medication	Block Placement	Dosing After Block Placement	Catheter Removal	Special Considerations
Heparin 5000 U SC BID	No contraindications although risk may be reduced when heparin injection is administered after the block	No contraindications	No contraindications	Concurrent medications affecting clotting system Check platelet count when administered >4 d
Heparin 5000 U SC TID	Insufficient evidence. Assess risk/benefits for each patient	Insufficient evidence	Insufficient evidence	Assess risk/benefits for each patient
Heparin infusion	Assess coagulation status. Delay placement for 6 h after heparin discontinued and normal coagulation achieved	Delay until 1 h after block placement	Assess coagulation status. Remove catheter 2–4 h after last heparin dose	Reheparinize 1 h after catheter removal Assess risks/benefits in event of bloody or difficult epidural placement
LMWH (thromboprophylaxis: once-daily dosing)	Delay 10–12 h after last dose	Delay until 6–8 h after block placement	Remove catheter 10–12 h after last dose	Administer 2 h after catheter removal Delay 24 h for traumatic epidural placement
LMWH (thromboprophylaxis: twice-daily dosing)	Delay at least 24 h after last dose	Delay 1st dose 6–8 h after block and 2nd dose no sooner than 24 h after 1st dose	Incompatible with indwelling epidural catheter	Administer 2 h after catheter removal. Delay 24 h for traumatic epidural placement
Therapeutic LMWH	Delay at least 24 h after last dose	Delay 24 h after block placement	Remove catheter before administration Incompatible with indwelling epidural catheter	Administer 2 h after catheter removal Delay 24 h for traumatic epidural
Warfarin (Coumadin)	Discontinue 4–5 d and normal INR before block placement	No recommendations	Remove catheter when INR <1.5	Monitor INR daily if warfarin started when epidural in place

Abbreviations: ASRA, American Society of Regional Anesthesia and Pain Medicine; BID, twice daily; INR, international normalized ratio; LMWH, low molecular weight heparin; SC, subcutaneous; TID, 3 times daily; U, units.

Data from Horlocker TT, Wedel DJ, Rowlingson JC, et al. Regional anesthesia in the patient receiving antithrombotic or thrombolytic therapy: American Society of Regional Anesthesia and Pain Medicine evidence-based guidelines (3rd edition). Reg Anesth Pain Med 2010;35(1):4-7.

Table 4
Neuraxial anesthesia and antiplatelet agents

Medication	Recommendations
NSAIDs	No contraindications
Clopidogrel (Plavix)	Discontinue 7 d before block placement
Tilclopidine (Ticlid)	Discontinue 14 d before block placement
Abciximab[a] (Reopro)	Discontinue 24–48 h until platelet aggregation normalized
Eptifibatide[a] (Integrilin) Tirofiban[a] (Aggrastat)	Discontinue 4–8 h until platelet aggregation normalized

Abbreviation: NSAIDs, nonsteroidal anti-inflammatory drugs.
[a] Group IIb/IIIa antagonists are contraindicated within 4 weeks of surgery.
Adapted from Horlocker TT, Wedel DJ, Rowlingson JC, et al. Regional anesthesia in the patient receiving antithrombotic or thrombolytic therapy: American Society of Regional Anesthesia and Pain Medicine evidence-based guidelines (3rd Edition). Reg Anesth Pain Med 2010;35(1):78–9; with permission.

commonly used agents. Opioids should be used cautiously in high-risk populations, including the elderly, obese, and those with obstructive or central sleep apnea.

Selective peripheral opioid antagonists, such as methylnaltrexone, may be suggested by the APMS to treat postoperative opioid-induced ileus and other side effects without reversing the analgesia. It is the authors' experience that many clinicians are unaware of the availability of this agent, so the APMS can play an important role in this regard. Other less serious but bothersome side effects of epidural opioids include pruritus, nausea and vomiting, and urinary retention. Treatments for these relatively common issues should be part of standard order sets.

The epidural infusion can be started in either the operating room or the postanesthesia care unit (PACU). Proper communication between the APMS and the anesthesia team prevents unnecessary repeat test doses and clarifies any intraoperative issues, such as hypotension or bleeding. Typical epidural solutions used at the authors' institution are listed in **Table 5**. It is important to not exceed the recommended allowable dosage of the local anesthetic. The infusion settings are typically titrated to patient satisfaction. Patients are monitored by APMS during the postoperative stay for pain scores, cardiovascular parameters, motor blockade, and proper functioning of the epidural. There is a small risk of catheter migration into the venous system or the subarachnoid space. Appropriate monitoring and vigilance by the APMS team can prevent many complications from occurring. Because epidural infusions often require periodic bolus doses, the round-the-clock availability of APMS nurses, in addition to residents or fellows, can facilitate the maintenance of analgesia.

CONTINUOUS PERIPHERAL NERVE BLOCKS
Potential Complications of Upper and Lower Extremity Nerve Blocks

CPNBs, both upper and lower extremity, improve postoperative analgesia, increase patient satisfaction, and enhance surgical outcomes and patient rehabilitation in comparison with opioid-based analgesia.[31–34] Patients receiving brachial plexus blockade for shoulder surgery are significantly less likely to have pain, nausea, and vomiting. In addition, PACU stays are shorter.[35] Perineural brachial plexus catheters, both inpatient and ambulatory, provide prolonged analgesia (up to 72 hours), faster resumption of physical therapy, less reliance on opioids, fewer sleep disturbances at home, and overall increased patient satisfaction at home.[36] Postoperative analgesia for lower extremity surgery may be achieved by a variety of peripheral nerve blocks (lumbar plexus

Table 5
Epidural solutions using continuous or patient-controlled epidural analgesia

	Continuous (mL/h)	PCEA		
		Demand (mL)	Lockout (min)	Continuous (mL/h)
0.125% bupivacaine	6–10 (thoracic) 10–16 (lumbar)	2	20	5–8
0.125% bupivacaine + 5 μg/mL fentanyl	6–10 (thoracic) 10–16 (lumbar)	2	10	5
0.125% bupivacaine + 5 μg/mL hydromorphone	6–10 (thoracic) 10–14 (lumbar)	2	20	5
0.125% bupivacaine + epinephrine 1:400,000	6–10 (thoracic) 10–16 (lumbar)	2	10	5
0.2% ropivacaine	6–10 (thoracic) 10–16 (lumbar)	2	20	5–8
0.2% ropivacaine + 5 μg/mL fentanyl	6–10 (thoracic) 10–16 (lumbar)	2	10	5
0.2% ropivacaine + 5 μg/mL hydromorphone	6–10 (thoracic) 10–16 (lumbar)	2	20	5
0.2% ropivacaine + epinephrine 1:400,000	6–10 (thoracic) 10–16 (lumbar)	2	10	5

Abbreviation: PCEA, patient-controlled epidural analgesia.

block, femoral nerve block, adductor canal block, and sciatic nerve block), which, unlike epidural analgesia, do not cause hypotension or urinary retention. Collectively, CPNBs provide analgesia superior to that of opioids and decrease their unwanted side effects.[37] However, CPNBs are not without side effects and risks (**Table 6**).

One of the more feared complications of peripheral nerve blocks is nerve injury; however, nerve injury is often temporary and the incidence is estimated at approximately 1 in 5000.[38] In a study of more than 7000 peripheral nerve blocks performed using a variety of techniques including ultrasound guidance, nerve stimulation, and a combination, 30 patients (0.5%) were referred for neurologic assessment; however, only 3 patients (0.04%) met the criteria for nerve injury related to peripheral nerve block.[39] While the exact mechanism of peripheral nerve injury following perineural blockade is unclear, patients with preexisting neuropathy, especially diabetics and those who have received neurotoxic chemotherapy, may be more susceptible.[40] It is imperative that the APMS team monitors for signs of nerve injury, especially persistent weakness, or paresthesias in the nerve block distribution following expected primary block resolution or CPNB discontinuation. Although permanent nerve injury is rare, as much as 8% to 10% of patients may experience transient paresthesia in the days to weeks following blockade.[39] If signs of nerve injury are observed, patient education and reassurance, in addition to neurologist referral, are recommended.

Although perineural catheters have a high rate of bacterial colonization ranging from 7.5% to 57%, localized inflammation is infrequent (0%–13.7%) and infection (0%–3.2%), abscess formation (0%–0.9%), and sepsis are rare.[36] The APMS team members must take an active role in monitoring CPNB sites for signs of infection, including erythema, drainage, and pain at the catheter insertion site. Typically, CPNBs are removed 48 to 72 hours following placement. Occasionally perineural catheters have remained in place for up to 7 to 10 days without incident at the authors'

Table 6
Indications and side effects/complications of peripheral nerve blocks

Peripheral Nerve Block	Indications	Complications and Side Effects

Interscalene block (roots/trunks)	Shoulder arthroscopy
	Rotator cuff repair
	Shoulder arthroplasty
	Fracture of humerus neck
		Complications:
		  Nerve injury
		  Unintended spinal/epidural injection
		  Hematoma
		  Pneumothorax (rare)
		Side effects:
		  Horner syndrome
		  Temporary phrenic nerve paralysis (100% incidence)
		  Temporary hoarseness/dysphagia

Supraclavicular block (divisions)	Total elbow replacement
	Ulnar nerve repair
	Hand surgery
		Complications:
		  Nerve injury
		  Hematoma
		  Pneumothorax
		Side effects:
		  Temporary phrenic nerve paralysis (50% incidence)

Infraclavicular/axillary block (cords/terminal nerves)	Total elbow replacement
	Carpal tunnel repair
	Hand/digit surgery
		Complications:
		  Nerve injury
		  Hematoma
		  Pneumothorax (rare)

Lumbar plexus block	THA
	ORIF of acetabular fracture
	TKA
	Quadriceps repair
		Complications:
		  Nerve injury
		  Hematoma (adhere to neuraxial anticoagulation guidelines)
		Side effects:
		  Unilateral sympathectomy/hypotension
		  Quadriceps weakness/fall risk

Femoral nerve block (FNB)	TKA
	ACL repair
	Quadriceps repair
	Adjuvant to sciatic block for foot/ankle surgery
		Complications:
		  Nerve injury
		  Hematoma
		  Infection
		Side effects
		  Quadriceps weakness/fall risk

Adductor canal block	TKA
	ACL repair
	Quadriceps repair
	Adjuvant to sciatic block for foot/ankle surgery
		Complications:
		  Nerve injury
		  Hematoma
		Side effects:
		  Quadriceps weakness/fall risk (possibly lower fall risk than femoral nerve block)

Sciatic nerve block	Labat approach:
	  Hamstring surgery
	  Adjuvant to FNB for TKA
	Popliteal approach:
	  Total ankle replacement
	  Foot/ankle surgery
	  Metatarsal amputation
		Complications:
		  Nerve injury
		  Hematoma
		Side effects:
		  Insensate extremity/fall risk

Abbreviations: ACL, anterior cruciate ligament; ORIF, open reduction internal fixation; THA, total hip arthroplasty; TKA, total knee arthroplasty.

institution, but a risk/benefit discussion should take place. However, as with any indwelling catheter, daily site inspection is mandated.

Secondary block failure, which may be defined as a partially or completely ineffective level of peripheral nerve blockade from a continuous catheter, must be considered when analgesia is inadequate following primary block resolution. The incidence has been estimated at 10% to 40%.[41] A 10-mL bolus of concentrated local anesthetic (eg, ropivacaine 0.5%) through the catheter can help determine if the catheter is in the proper location. If analgesia is still inadequate, the APMS and the patient should discuss whether another primary block is desired and practical. If the decision is made to repeat the block, the patient should be brought to the perioperative area and monitored according to usual standards, and stay in the PACU if sedation is given. Bedside blocks on unmonitored wards are generally not recommended, as conditions are not ideal and resuscitation equipment may not be readily available. APMS team members must be familiar with the presentations of local anesthetic systemic toxicity and its treatment, including the use of lipid rescue therapy. CPNBs should always be aspirated before the injection of a bolus, as catheters can migrate and become intravascular.

Accidental catheter removal is another potential concern with CPNBs. The incidence appears to be low (1%), however, when both a skin sealant and an epidural catheter locking device are used, which Fredrickson and colleagues[42] showed in a group of 300 patients who received ambulatory interscalene catheters. The authors use a similar technique. Catheter kinking and looping are rare, and may be prevented by threading superficial catheters (brachial plexus) 3 cm past the needle tip and deeper catheters (femoral and sciatic) 5 to 10 cm beyond the needle tip.[43] Care must be taken to ensure that perineural catheters are safely removed and intact. If the provider feels tension on removal, patient repositioning and gentle traction may be necessary. The need for surgical removal of perineural catheters is very rare. Catheter site leakage is a common complaint among patients. Often this occurs in superficial catheters (eg, interscalene) as the local anesthetic is being infused just below the skin. Patient reassurance and reinforcement with a gauze dressing may be necessary.

Monitoring for Falls in Patients with Lower Extremity Blockade

CPNBs may cause muscle weakness that may interfere with rehabilitation and increase the risk of falls. Patients and staff must be educated on the concerns of an insensate lower extremity and the risk of falls associated with lower extremity peripheral nerve blockade. The literature is inconclusive with regard to fall risk, as one study suggested a causal relationship between lower extremity peripheral blockade for total joint arthroplasty and falls,[44] whereas another found no difference.[45] In one study, 29% of patients who received a femoral nerve block (FNB) had knee buckling secondary to decreased quadriceps strength, compared with 3% of controls.[46] The adductor canal block has become increasingly popular as an alternative to the FNB for knee surgery. It causes less quadriceps weakness than an FNB[47] and may provide similar analgesia.[48] However, APMS team members should understand that quadriceps weakness can still occur, and educate patients and their care providers about this. Falls attributed to perineural blockade may be the result of sensory loss, motor weakness, impaired proprioception, or a combination.[44]

The APMS has an integral role in educating patients and nursing staff on the risk of falls and the need for assistance with ambulation in patients with CPNBs of the lower extremity. Fall precautions must be clearly delineated. In addition, the lowest dose possible of local anesthetic should be administered via the catheter to minimize motor block while still achieving satisfactory analgesia. It is also worth mentioning that injection of boluses through the catheter, especially using high concentrations of local anesthetic, can exacerbate muscle weakness.

The Role of Local Anesthetic Additives in Perineural Analgesia

In recent years, much focus has been directed on determining effective local anesthetic additives for prolonging postoperative perineural analgesia. Continuous catheters may be cumbersome, may leak, or may fail because of dislodgment, and may be expensive and more time-consuming to place. In addition, the location of the surgical field may prohibit preoperative CPNB placement.

Familiarity with frequently used additives is imperative for APMS team members, as additives may significantly prolong not only sensory but also motor blockade. Dexmedetomidine, a potent α2-agonist, has shown promise as a perineural local anesthetic additive, and may decrease local anesthetic-induced perineural inflammation.[49] Buprenorphine, a partial μ-receptor opioid agonist, has shown a significant increase in block duration (up to 4 times that of local anesthetic alone). However, the results are more pronounced for upper extremity blockade.[50,51] Dexamethasone has also shown significant promise as a perineural local anesthetic additive, significantly prolonging sensory and motor block duration.[52] APMS nurses should be educated on expected primary block durations with additives so that they can anticipate the return of motor function in patients with a CPNB. In turn, they can educate surgeons and others on the expected return of motor function if additives have been used in peripheral nerve blocks.

The Role of the Acute Pain Management Service in an Ambulatory Continuous Perineural Catheter Service

Recent evidence suggests that ambulatory CPNBs improve analgesia, reduce sleep disturbances, decrease opioid consumption and related side effects, and enhance patient satisfaction.[53] Patient selection is critical to the success of ambulatory CPNBs. Some contraindications include severe hepatic or renal insufficiency and, in the case of brachial plexus blockade, severe respiratory impairment. Serious consideration should be given to the maturity level and comprehension of the patients. Patients with generalized anxiety disorder or panic disorder may be poor candidates.

Preoperative instructions can help minimize confusion, as the effects of anesthesia may make postoperative instructions difficult to remember. Both verbal and written instructions must be provided, specifically reviewing the infusion pump details, analgesic expectations with regard to primary block resolution, catheter site care, insensate limb protection precautions, fall risks, breakthrough pain instructions, care for catheter site leakage, signs of local anesthetic toxicity and need for emergency care, and catheter removal instructions. In addition, clear 24-hour contact information must be provided, and a system must be in place to enable the patient to contact the APMS with questions. All members of the APMS must be educated on CPNB complications, commonly asked questions, and when to recognize an emergency, such as local anesthetic systemic toxicity. The authors recommend contacting each patient with an ambulatory CPNB daily via a telephone follow-up interview and documenting each encounter. In addition, regarding infusions the authors use a ropivacaine 0.2% infusion at 6 to 8 mL/h for brachial plexus catheters and 8 to 10 mL/h for lower extremity catheters.

SUMMARY

Delivery of a high-quality APMS presents many challenges. An organized approach with dedicated, trained individuals is critical. An institutional commitment is mandatory to assure a hospital-wide, integrated approach. Organization tools improve efficiency and safety while improving quality. Health care is increasingly driven by patient satisfaction, and pain management is a significant driver for patient satisfaction. As anesthesiologists expand their role outside the operating room, acute pain management provides an opportunity to provide an added-value service in a competitive health care market.

REFERENCES

1. Kehlet H, Morgensen T. Hospital stay of 2 days after open sigmoidectomy with a multimodal rehabilitation programme. Br J Surg 1999;86:227–30.
2. Elia N, Lysakowski C, Tramer MR. Does multimodal analgesia with acetaminophen, nonsteroidal antiinflammatory drugs, or selective cyclooxygenase-2 inhibitors and patient-controlled analgesia morphine offer advantages over morphine alone? Anesthesiology 2005;103:1296–304.
3. Hurley RW, Cohen SP, Williams KA, et al. The analgesic effects of perioperative gabapentin on postoperative pain: a meta-analysis. Reg Anesth Pain Med 2006; 31:237–47.
4. Zhang J, Ho KY, Wang Y. Efficacy of pregabalin in acute postoperative pain: a meta-analysis. Br J Anaesth 2011;106:454–62.
5. Afridi SK, Giffin NJ, Kaube H, et al. A randomized controlled trial of intranasal ketamine in migraine with prolonged aura. Neurology 2013;80:642–7.
6. Date DF, Sanfey H, Mellinger J, et al. Handoffs in general surgery residency, an observation of intern and senior residents. Am J Surg 2013;206:693–7.
7. Ballantyne JC, Carr DB, Chalmers TC, et al. Postoperative patient-controlled analgesia: meta-analyses of initial randomized control trials. J Clin Anesth 1993;5:182–93.
8. Parker RK, Holtmann B, White PF. Patient-controlled analgesia: does a concurrent opioid infusion improve pain management after surgery? JAMA 1991;266:1947–52.
9. White PF. Use of patient-controlled analgesia for management of acute pain. JAMA 1988;259:243–7.
10. White PF. Mishaps with patient-controlled analgesia. Anesthesiology 1987;66: 81–3.
11. Hudson TJ, Edlung MJ, Steffick DE, et al. Epidemiology of regular opioid use: results from a national, population-based survey. J Pain Symptom Manage 2008;36:280–8.
12. Mazer-Amirshahi M, Mullins PM, Rasooly I, et al. Rising opioid prescribing in adult U.S. emergency department visits: 2001-2010. Acad Emerg Med 2014; 21:236–43.
13. Chazan S, Ekstein MP, Marouani N, et al. Ketamine for acute and subacute pain in opioid-tolerant patients. J Opioid Manag 2008;4:173–80.
14. Marcucci C, Fudin J, Thomas P, et al. A new pattern of buprenorphine misuse may complicate perioperative pain control. Anesth Analg 2009;108:1996–7.
15. Chen KY, Chen L, Mao J. Buprenorphine-naloxone therapy in pain management. Anesthesiology 2014;120:1262–74.
16. Bryson EO. The perioperative management of patients maintained on medications used to manage opioid addiction. Curr Opin Anaesthesiol 2014;27:359–64.
17. Block BM, Liu SS, Rowlingson AJ, et al. Efficacy of postoperative epidural analgesia: a meta-analysis. JAMA 2003;290:2455–63.
18. Wu C, Cohen SR, Richman JM, et al. Efficacy of postoperative patient-controlled and continuous infusion epidural analgesia versus intravenous patient-controlled analgesia with opioids. Anesthesiology 2005;103:1079–88.

19. Ballantyne JC, Carr DB, deFerranti S, et al. The comparative effects of postoperative analgesic therapies on pulmonary outcomes: cumulative meta-analyses of randomized, controlled trials. Anesth Analg 1998;86:598–612.
20. Carli F, Trudel JL, Belliveau P. The effect of intraoperative thoracic epidural anesthesia and postoperative analgesia on bowel function after colorectal surgery: a prospective, randomized trial. Dis Colon Rectum 2001;44:1083–9.
21. Wijeysunderat DN, Beattie WS, Austin PC, et al. Epidural anaesthesia and survival after intermediate to high risk non-cardiac surgery: a population-based cohort study. Lancet 2008;372:562–9.
22. Horlocker TT, Wedel DJ, Rowlingson JC, et al. Regional anesthesia in the patient receiving antithrombotic or thrombolytic therapy: American Society of Regional Anesthesia and Pain Medicine Evidence-Based Guidelines (Third Edition). Reg Anesth Pain Med 2010;35(1):64–101.
23. Niemi G, Breivik H. Adrenaline markedly improves thoracic epidural analgesia produced by a low-dose infusion of bupivacaine, fentanyl and adrenaline after major surgery. A randomized double-blind, cross-over study with and without adrenaline. Acta Anaesthesiol Scand 1998;42:897–909.
24. Forster JG, Rosenberg PH. Small dose of clonidine mixed with low-dose ropivacaine and fentanyl for epidural analgesia after total knee arthroplasty. Br J Anaesth 2004;93:670–7.
25. Chia YY, Liu K, Liu YC, et al. Adding ketamine in a multimodal patient-controlled epidural regimen reduces postoperative pain and analgesic consumption. Anesth Analg 1998;86:1245–9.
26. Kampe S, Weigand C, Kaufmann J, et al. Postoperative analgesia with no motor block by continuous epidural infusion of ropivacaine 0.1% and sufentanil after total hip replacement. Anesth Analg 1999;89:395–8.
27. Wieblack A, Brodneer G, Van Aken H. The effects of adding sufentanil to bupivacaine postoperative patient-controlled epidural analgesia. Anesth Analg 1997;85:124–9.
28. Mourisse J, Hasenbos MA, Gielen MJ, et al. Epidural bupivacaine, sufentanil or the combination for post-thoracotomy pain. Acta Anaesthesiol Scand 1992;36:70–4.
29. Crews JC, Hord AH, Denson DD, et al. A comparison of the analgesic efficacy of 0.25% levobupivacaine combined with 0.005% morphine, 0.25% levobupivacaine alone, or 0.005% morphine alone for the management of postoperative pain in patients undergoing major abdominal surgery. Anesth Analg 1999;89:1504–9.
30. Maalouf DB, Liu SS. Clinical applications of epidural analgesia. In: Sinatra RS, de Leon-Casasola OA, Ginsberg B, et al, editors. Acute pain management. New York: Cambridge University Press; 2009. p. 114–43.
31. Borgeat A, Tewes E, Biasca N, et al. Patient-controlled interscalene analgesia with ropivacaine after major shoulder surgery: PCIA vs PCA. Br J Anaesth 1998;81:603–5.
32. Borgeat A, Schappi B, Biasca N, et al. Patient-controlled analgesia after major shoulder surgery: patient-controlled interscalene analgesia versus patient-controlled analgesia. Anesthesiology 1997;87:1343–7.
33. Capdevila X, Barthelet Y, Biboulet P, et al. Effects of perioperative analgesic technique on the surgical outcome and duration of rehabilitation after major knee surgery. Anesthesiology 1999;91:8–15.
34. Singelyn FJ, Deyaett M, Jotis D, et al. Effects of intravenous patient-controlled analgesia and continuous three-in-one block on postoperative pain and knee rehabilitation after unilateral total knee arthroplasty. Anesth Analg 1998;87:88–92.

35. Hadzic A, Williams BA, Karaca PE, et al. For outpatient rotator cuff surgery, nerve block anesthesia provides superior same-day recovery over general anesthesia. Anesthesiology 2005;102(5):1001–7.

36. Ilfeld BM. Continuous peripheral nerve blocks: a review of the published evidence. Anesth Analg 2011;113(4):904–25.

37. Richman JM, Liu SS, Courpas G, et al. Does continuous peripheral nerve block provide superior pain control to opioids? A meta-analysis. Anesth Analg 2006; 102(1):248–57.

38. Fowler SJ, Symons J, Sabato S, et al. Epidural analgesia compared with peripheral nerve blockade after major knee surgery: a systematic review and meta-analysis of randomized trials. Br J Anaesth 2008;100(2):154–64.

39. Jeng CL, Torrillo TM, Rosenblatt MA. Complications of peripheral nerve blocks. Br J Anaesth 2010;105(S1):i97–107.

40. Kroin JS, Buvanendran A, Williams DK, et al. Local anesthetic sciatic nerve block and nerve fiber damage in diabetic rats. Reg Anesth Pain Med 2010; 35:343–50.

41. Salinas FV. Location, location, location: continuous peripheral nerve blocks and stimulating catheters. Reg Anesth Pain Med 2003;28:79–82.

42. Fredrickson MJ, Ball CM, Dalgleish AJ. Successful continuous interscalene analgesia for ambulatory shoulder surgery in a private practice setting. Reg Anesth Pain Med 2008;33:122–8.

43. Rudd K, Hall PJ. Knotted femoral nerve catheter. Anaesth Intensive Care 2004; 32:282–3.

44. Ilfeld BM, Duke KB, Donohue MC. The association between lower extremity continuous peripheral nerve blocks and patient falls after knee and hip arthroplasty. Anesth Analg 2010;111:1552–4.

45. Chelly JE, Ghisi D, Fanelli A. Continuous peripheral nerve blocks in acute pain management. Br J Anaesth 2010;105(S1):i86–96.

46. YaDeau JT, Cahill JB, Zawadsky MW, et al. The effects of femoral nerve blockade in conjunction with epidural analgesia after total knee arthroplasty. Anesth Analg 2005;101:891–5.

47. Kwofie MK, Shastri UD, Gadsen JC, et al. The effects of ultrasound-guided adductor canal block versus femoral nerve block on quadriceps strength and fall risk: a blinded, randomized trial of volunteers. Reg Anesth Pain Med 2013; 38:321–5.

48. Kim DH, Lin Y, Goytizolo EA, et al. Adductor canal block versus femoral nerve block for total knee arthroplasty. Anesthesiology 2014;120:540–50.

49. Marhofer D, Kettner SC, Marhofer P, et al. Dexmedetomidine as an adjuvant to ropivacaine prolongs peripheral nerve block: a volunteer study. Br J Anaesth 2013;110(3):438–42.

50. Candido KD, Winnie AP, Ghaleb AH, et al. Buprenorphine added to the local anesthetic for axillary brachial plexus block prolongs postoperative analgesia. Reg Anesth Pain Med 2002;27:162–7.

51. Candido KD, Hennes J, Gonzalez S, et al. Buprenorphine enhances and prolongs the postoperative analgesic effect of bupivacaine in patients receiving infragluteal sciatic nerve block. Anesthesiology 2010;113(6):1419–26.

52. Cummings KC, Napierkowski DE, Parra-Sanchez I, et al. Effect of dexamethasone on the duration of interscalene nerve blocks with ropivacaine or bupivacaine. Br J Anaesth 2011;107(3):446–53.

53. Ilfeld BM, Enneking FK. Continuous peripheral nerve blocks at home: a review. Anesth Analg 2004;100:1822–33.

Setting Up an Ambulatory Regional Anesthesia Program for Orthopedic Surgery

Danielle B. Ludwin, MD

KEYWORDS

- Ambulatory anesthesia • Regional anesthesia • Peripheral nerve block • Efficiency
- Quality improvement • Patient satisfaction • Optimizing perineural analgesia
- Systems-based improvement

KEY POINTS

- Setting up an ambulatory regional anesthesia program for orthopedic surgery requires a multidisciplinary approach among anesthesiologists, surgeons, and nurses with all aspects of perioperative care considered.
- Regional anesthesia has distinct advantages in the orthopedic population by optimizing pain control and minimizing postoperative nausea and vomiting.
- To provide effective regional anesthesia, anesthesiologists need to consider a streamlined approach whereby peripheral nerve blocks can be placed expeditiously and post anesthesia care unit time can be minimized.
- A system needs to be in place for managing complications perioperatively.

INTRODUCTION

Ambulatory anesthesia case volume is increasing as more complex procedures are being transferred to the outpatient setting in efforts to contain costs and promote efficiency. The number of ambulatory surgeries reported by Colorado, New Jersey, and New York grew from 900,000 to 2,720,834 between 1988 and 2008.[1] Regional anesthesia complements this shift to ambulatory anesthesia by using targeted anesthesia methods that can minimize opioid requirements, reduce anesthetic side effects, promote earlier discharge, and achieve higher patient satisfaction.

POTENTIAL ADVANTAGES OF REGIONAL ANESTHESIA
Regional Anesthesia Optimizes Analgesia

Regional anesthesia allows site-specific anesthesia and analgesia, reducing and possibly eliminating the need for perioperative opioids and their related side effects.

Disclosure: None.
Division of Regional and Orthopedic Anesthesia, Department of Anesthesiology, Columbia University College of Physicians & Surgeons, 630 West 168th Street, P & S Box 46, New York, NY 10032, USA
E-mail address: dl2453@cumc.columbia.edu

Anesthesiology Clin 32 (2014) 911–921
http://dx.doi.org/10.1016/j.anclin.2014.08.011   **anesthesiology.theclinics.com**

Local anesthetics have been shown to decrease postoperative pain.[2] Multiple meta-analyses have established that regional anesthesia provides better quality analgesia than systemic opioids. Continuous perineural local anesthetic infusions can improve analgesia for up to 48 hours after surgery compared with opioids.[3–5] Compared with single-injection peripheral nerve blockade, continuous peripheral nerve blockade results in decreased pain scores up to 48 hours postoperatively, decreased opioid use, decreased nausea, and improved patient satisfaction scores.[6]

Regional Anesthesia Decreases Postoperative Nausea and Vomiting

Postoperative nausea and vomiting (PONV) was identified as the number one postoperative complaint in a prospective interview study of more than 12,000 patients, with 13.9% of patients reporting PONV.[7] Other studies have found patients are willing to pay $17 to $100 in out-of-pocket costs for PONV treatment.[8,9] In the Society for Ambulatory Anesthesia guidelines on the management of PONV published in 2014, regional anesthesia is recommended to avoid general anesthesia and thus reduce the risk of PONV.[10]

Regional Anesthesia Can Prevent Unanticipated Admissions and Lead to Earlier Discharge

Unanticipated inpatient admissions are often attributed to pain and PONV after ambulatory surgery. Based on data from the 2006 National Survey of Ambulatory Surgery, unexpected ambulatory admission rates were 0.6% for knee procedures and 4.8% after shoulder surgery.[11] Successful regional anesthesia management can circumvent these issues.[12]

Several studies have shown decreased time to home discharge using peripheral nerve blockade over general anesthesia for patients undergoing interscalene block (ISB), infraclavicular, and axillary block for upper extremity procedures.[13–18] Patients receiving short-acting lumbar plexus and sciatic nerve blocks for outpatient knee surgery had faster discharge times as well as a greater likelihood of post anesthesia care unit (PACU) bypass.[19]

Regional Anesthesia Can Increase Efficiency

Regional anesthesia can optimize outcomes and improve operating room efficiency. A clinical pathway for anterior cruciate ligament reconstruction surgery incorporating regional anesthesia was implemented at an ambulatory surgery center in a teaching hospital in Pittsburgh. The pathway was created with multidisciplinary input from anesthesiologists, surgeons, perioperative nurses, physical therapists, and nursing administrators. Executing this clinical algorithm positively resulted in decreased pharmacy and materials cost, decreased anesthesia controlled time (time patient in room to start of positioning and prepping), decreased surgeon controlled times, a decrease in the number of required nursing interventions for common postoperative conditions, and decreased unexpected admissions for nausea, vomiting, and pain. The pathway was associated negatively with an increase in turnover time. Implementing these changes within clinical pathways provides an opportunity to maximize systems and processes, and to identify potential areas for improvement as well as opportunities to correct deficiencies.[20]

Another study on efficiency reviewed arthroscopic shoulder surgery anesthesia. ISB was shown to improve anesthesia-related workflow times over general anesthesia. The ISB group had a PACU time of 45 minutes, compared with 70 minutes for the general anesthesia group.[21]

Regional Anesthesia Can Improve Patient Satisfaction

Patient satisfaction is an important component of optimizing the perioperative experience. Many patients prefer to receive regional anesthesia instead of general anesthesia, and some patients may choose hospitals or ambulatory settings where regional anesthesia is offered as an option. In a prospective interview study, patient satisfaction was increased by the use of regional anesthesia over general anesthesia.[7] Patients surveyed from the international registry of regional anesthesia reported that approximately 95% would have a repeat peripheral nerve block, and 90% of patients were satisfied or completely satisfied with the education provided about the block.[22]

Surgeons May Prefer Regional Anesthesia

Involving orthopedic surgeons in the planning process for a new ambulatory regional anesthesia program is critical. An interdisciplinary approach should be discussed to minimize case delays, formulate a plan for assessment of blocks with a backup management plan for any failed blocks, and create a system for managing complications.[23] Additionally, surgeons need to have realistic expectations regarding what regional anesthesia can provide (ie, a patient with a popliteal sciatic nerve block for lower extremity surgery will still have partial motor function of the lower extremity).

PRACTICAL DETAILS FOR ORGANIZING AN AMBULATORY REGIONAL ANESTHESIA SERVICE
Patient Education and Screening

Setting up expectations and goals for patients is critical to the success of an ambulatory regional anesthesia service. Preoperative counseling allows the patient to seek further information and clarify questions ahead of time. Thorough preoperative education can expedite block placement on the day of surgery and minimize unnecessary stress for patients by allowing them to be better educated and more informed. Patients who were surveyed about their experiences after a peripheral nerve block were more likely to report dissatisfaction if they felt that not enough information had been provided or they experienced a poor professional interaction with their anesthesiologist.[22]

Print or digital educational materials about regional anesthesia should be made available to the patient before their surgery. Patients can be educated about regional anesthesia options by their surgeon in a preoperative visit, at a preanesthesia clinic, or from the nursing or anesthesiology team via a phone call the night before surgery. Beyond discussing regional anesthesia, patients can be educated about the entire perioperative experience. Screening patients preoperatively creates an opportunity to optimize medical conditions to avoid day of surgery delays and/or cancellations and to assess the appropriateness of patients for outpatient surgery.[24] During the admissions process on the day of surgery, candidates for regional anesthesia should ideally be fast tracked to minimize delays.

Proper selection of patients for ambulatory regional anesthesia is an important consideration. Patients should be carefully screened if ambulatory perineural catheters are planned for procedures that ordinarily require inpatient admission. Perineural catheter candidates should have a solid support system, have the ability to be compliant with instructions, and be within a reasonable distance from a hospital should they require medical attention after discharge. Patients with significant comorbidities, such as pulmonary, cardiac, renal, hepatic, and coagulopathic disease, need to undergo a careful risk–benefit assessment.[25]

Resources Including Equipment and Personnel

Practical considerations for an ambulatory orthopedic regional anesthesia service include having skilled practitioners to increase efficiency and likelihood of regional anesthesia success. Specialized teams who have standardized practices and a subspecialty knowledge base have been shown to have stronger working relationships with surgical and nursing colleagues.[26] Forming a multidisciplinary team allows the creation of clinical pathways, which can optimize the perioperative experience on an institution-specific level.[27] For practices initiating a new ambulatory regional orthopedic service, consider a pilot program with American Society of Anesthesiologists class I and II patients. This exercise provides the opportunity to smooth out unforeseen organizational challenges and introduce necessary changes before a formal, full-service rollout.

In addition to anesthesiology staff, the regional anesthesia team may be composed of regional anesthesiology and acute pain medicine fellows, residents, and nurses. Specifically trained nurses dedicated to the perioperative care of patients undergoing regional anesthesia procedures (sometimes referred to as "block" nurses) may improve efficiency and may increase patient safety by ensuring that the preblock checklist is followed, including correct patient, site, and laterality confirmation.[28]

Performing regional anesthesia requires capital purchases including nerve stimulators and/or ultrasound machines. Supplies are typically organized in a regional anesthesia "block cart." If perineural catheters are utilized, then infusion devices may be required. Resuscitation equipment, including airway instrumentation, lipid emulsion, and an algorithm for the management of local anesthetic systemic toxicity, should be immediately available.[29]

Proper documentation of perineural blockade is critical.[30] The procedure note or anesthesia/nursing record should include the patient's vital signs, level of sedation, drugs administered, cleansing solution, patient position, needle used with length and gauge, use of nerve stimulator, ultrasound or paresthesia technique, injectate type and dose, any adjuvants used, presence or absence of blood aspirated, and pain or resistance to injection.[31] All patients must undergo a history taking and physical examination with particular attention to any underlying neuropathy, coagulation issues, or extensive comorbidities that may influence whether regional anesthesia is an appropriate technique.

Techniques for Block Placement

Ultrasound guidance, landmark based (eg, nerve stimulation or paresthesia seeking), or a combined approach are most commonly used for nerve localization during perineural blockade. Excellent outcomes have been reported for all of these techniques, and the choice of technique depends on practitioner experience as well as available equipment. For the nerve stimulation technique, the use of a specialized insulated stimulating needle is recommended.

Local anesthetic selection for peripheral nerve blockade depends on the intended duration of block. Common local anesthetic agents include mepivacaine 1.5% with expected duration of 2 to 5 hours and ropivacaine 0.5% or bupivacaine 0.5% with expected durations of 10 to 14 hours.[32] Duration of peripheral nerve blockade depends on the dose of local anesthetic used, presence of adjuvants, and the location of the block, with less vascular areas lasting longer.[32] Clonidine, when added to local anesthetic solutions for peripheral nerve block, has been shown to increase block duration by about 2 hours.[33] The addition of dexamethasone results in a variable prolongation of analgesia and motor block after peripheral nerve blockade from 12 to 22 hours.[34] A recent study compared ISB with perineural ropivacaine, perineural ropivacaine, and dexamethasone, and perineural ropivacaine and systemic dexamethasone. The ropivacaine-only group had a sensory block duration of 757 minutes, which was significantly shorter than the duration of sensory blocks in both dexamethasone groups. The duration of sensory block was 1405 minutes in the intravenous dexamethasone group and was 1275 minutes for perineural dexamethasone.[35] Further studies are needed to determine the efficacy of perineural versus IV dexamethasone for block prolongation.

Ambulatory Orthopedic Procedures Amenable to Perineural Blockade

Most orthopedic procedures are amenable to perineural blockade (**Table 1**). Appropriate selection of cases is important to improve patient and surgeon satisfaction. Active discussion should take place preoperatively between the anesthesiology and surgical teams to clarify which procedures may be suitable for perineural blockade. For example, for carpal tunnel surgery, some orthopedic surgeons may prefer to do their own local anesthetic injection. For more invasive extremity surgeries, surgeons may be concerned that a perineural block may mask the development of compartment syndrome postoperatively. These nuanced situations need to be discussed on a case-by-case basis and resolved collaboratively before the performance of a regional anesthetic technique.

Models of Practice

There are several models of practice for setting up an ambulatory orthopedic regional anesthesia service. One model involves a block area, which may be located in a preoperative holding area or in a PACU. This area should be equipped with beds, standard monitors (American Society of Anesthesiologists), resuscitation equipment

Table 1	
Common ambulatory orthopedic peripheral nerve blocks	
Block[a,b]	**Indications**
Upper extremity	
Interscalene	Shoulder surgery
Supraclavicular	Most upper extremity procedures, for shoulder surgery prioritize superior trunks, for hand surgery prioritize "corner pocket" (where plexus, subclavian artery and first rib meet)[49]
Infraclavicular	Elbow, Forearm and Hand Surgery
Axillary	Elbow, Forearm and Hand Surgery
Lower extremity	
Lumbar plexus	Hip, knee, or foot surgery
Femoral	Thigh, knee, or foot (medial) surgery
Saphenous (adductor canal)	Knee, or foot (medial) surgery
Sciatic	Hip, knee, foot or ankle surgery

[a] Peripheral nerve blocks are typically performed with 20–40 mL of local anesthetic taking into consideration the patient's weight and total volume of local anesthetic planned.
[b] Local anesthetics used include 2% lidocaine, 1.5% mepivacaine, 0.2%–0.75% ropivacaine, and 0.25%–0.5% bupivacaine depending on desired onset and duration of block and if the block is being used for anesthetic or analgesic purposes. Higher concentrations are used for anesthetic dosing, lower concentrations for analgesic dosing.

including lipid emulsion, and regional anesthesia supplies.[30] Having a separate block area can permit additional teaching with less time pressure to perform the block. Peripheral nerve blockade can be thoroughly assessed before entering the operating room, and supplementation can be provided if necessary. Alternatively, blocks can be placed in the operating room immediately preceding surgery, immediately after the surgery, or in the PACU. The advantages of placing blocks before surgery include decreasing intraoperative anesthetic and opioid analgesic requirements, thus optimizing perioperative pain management and decreasing opioid-related side effects.[36]

Some practices have incorporated a hybrid model, which involves using a "swing" or induction room to decrease nonoperative time, defined as time from skin closure to skin incision for the next case. Using an induction room was found to increase throughput 33% with 5.6 cases being done in an average day versus 4.2 cases. The swing room was also used postoperatively, allowing an increase in PACU bypass rates (60% vs 0% for control patients), less postoperative opioid use (20% vs 82%), and decreased treatment required for PONV (2% vs 20%).[37] The optimal use of an induction room or block area requires a separate anesthesiology team or parallel processing model with part of the operating room team transporting the previous patient to the recovery room while the rest of the team prepares the room for turnover and gets the next patient ready in the induction room. This has been shown to decrease induction time and turnover time for cases done under local anesthesia.[38]

When considering integrating a block room into clinical practice, anesthesiologists need to determine staffing costs, space, equipment needed, and expected case volume. This will allow them to determine whether or not the block room will run efficiently and be cost effective.

Multimodal Approach and Clinical Pathways

In addition to setting up a highly efficient ambulatory orthopedic regional anesthesia service, a multimodal approach should be considered to further optimize perioperative analgesia and minimize opioid-related side effects. This can be accomplished through the use of systemic adjuvants, including nonsteroidal antiinflammatory drugs, acetaminophen, N-methyl D-aspartate antagonists (eg, ketamine), opioids, and calcium channel antagonists (eg, gabapentin and pregabalin).[39]

PONV-sparing techniques using regional anesthesia, avoiding nitrous oxide and volatile anesthetics, minimizing intraoperative and postoperative opioids, and maintaining adequate hydration should be considered for all patients. Patients at greater risk (females, nonsmokers, history of PONV, specific types of surgery) should have a PONV-sparing anesthetic approach utilizing more than 2 interventions that can include a 5-HT3 antagonist, dexamethasone, propofol anesthesia, acupuncture, or a scopolamine patch.[10]

Beyond the use of multimodal drug therapy, clinical pathways can enhance recovery protocols and integrate anesthesiology, surgical, nursing, and physical therapy goals. Staff at a large university hospital in Germany implemented a quality postoperative pain management system using a numerical rating scale that would trigger a nurse- or physician-based intervention as well as specific suggestions for PONV prophylaxis and treatment. Prospective surveys demonstrated a 25% to 30% decrease in pain after the intervention, a decrease in nausea from 40% to 17%, a decrease in vomiting from 25% to 11% on the day of discharge, and a decrease in fatigue from 76% to 30%.[40]

Postoperative Considerations

Postoperative management of patients who receive perineural blockade must include patient education about side effects of the block. Patients need to understand the limitations of their peripheral nerve blockade (ie, a patient with major foot surgery who receives a popliteal sciatic nerve block may have pain along the medial aspect of the ankle secondary to an unblocked saphenous nerve). Treatment includes a saphenous nerve block or using opioids and/or adjuvants for pain control. Patients also need to be informed as to when they can expect their nerve block to wear off and when they should start to take prescribed opioids as needed. It is often recommended that patients initiate oral opioid medication before peripheral nerve blockade regression to avoid a sudden and severe analgesic gap.

Patients need to be counseled that their extremity will be numb and may be subject to inadvertent injury. Therefore, no sharp objects should be near the extremity nor should the extremity be exposed to extreme heat or cold. They should have a caretaker who can assist them while they have an insensate extremity. A plan with the health care team should be established to determine whom the patient can contact if their pain control becomes inadequate after discharge. In rare cases, readmission may be necessary.

Patients need to be aware of site-specific complications. For brachial plexus blockade, this includes diaphragmatic paralysis of the affected side that manifests as the inability to take a deep breath using the accessory muscles of inspiration. Patients can have hoarseness if their recurrent laryngeal nerve has been blocked, and they can have a Horner's syndrome (ptosis, miosis, anhydriosis) from blockade of the cervical sympathetic chain. These side effects should resolve as the peripheral nerve blockade dissipates. Pneumothorax is also a rare risk for upper extremity peripheral nerve block, particularly with supraclavicular blocks.[41,42] Patients with new-onset pleuritic chest pain or decreased breath sounds on one side should be evaluated for a pneumothorax with a chest x-ray or ultrasonography.[43]

Lower extremity peripheral nerve blocks with lumbar plexus, femoral, or sciatic blocks can produce muscle weakness that may predispose patients to falls. Patients need to receive clear instructions and be educated about the risk of falls. If appropriate, patients should be taught to use crutches or a walker for mobilization. A knee immobilizer can be used to prevent quadriceps buckling. Patients should ambulate with assistance as needed. Patients should be counseled on all of these issues as applicable, and written instructions should be provided.[44]

A clear plan for determination of discharge readiness is an important postoperative consideration. The set of criteria used for PACU bypass and/or discharge can have significant implications for efficiency. Thus, patients who receive regional anesthesia may benefit from discharge criteria modified to account for peripheral nerve blockade. For example, having an insensate extremity, while typically accounting for a low score on standardized discharge criteria, does not apply to patients who undergo a peripheral nerve block.

WAKE discharge criteria have been developed and validated and may be more suitable for fast tracking patients who have received a regional anesthetic.[45,46] Scoring criteria include movement, blood pressure in relation to preoperative baseline blood pressure, level of consciousness, respiratory effort, and oxygen saturation. The WAKE score has "Zero Tolerance Criteria" that include pain that is not appropriately adjusted to the patients' baseline pain scores and a patient's complaint of PONV, shivering, pruritus, lightheadedness, or hypotension while sitting. Under these circumstances, the patient will not meet WAKE score phase I bypass criteria, thus decreasing the risk that patients may be fast tracked while still requiring significant nursing interventions.[45,46] The anesthesiology team needs to evaluate PACU patients using predefined criteria for suitability of discharge.

Table 2
Sample discharge instructions for peripheral nerve catheters

Instruction	Explanation
Protect your extremity	Avoid hot or cold temperatures near your numb arm or leg. Elevate the limb.
Catheter site	Some leaking at the site is normal. If there are large amounts of leakage or the catheter is disconnected, call the anesthesia service. Do not pull on the catheter. Do not get the dressing wet. If the site looks inflamed, red, painful or swollen call the anesthesiology service.
Local anesthesia toxicity signs	If the patient experiences numb lips, metallic taste in the mouth, ringing in the ears, dizziness, confusion, sleepiness, increased anxiety, shortness of breath, seizures or palpitations, turn off the catheter and call the anesthesiology service immediately.
Compartment syndrome signs	If the patient experiences significant pain in a previously numb extremity or the extremity changes color, turn off the catheter and call the surgery service immediately.
Removing the catheter	Wait until the patient can feel the limb, take off the dressing, slide the catheter out, and confirm tip. If any resistance or pain or numbness while removing the catheter, stop and call the anesthesiology service.
Specific pump instructions	Instructions on how to use bolus feature if prescribed, how to shut off pump, and contact information for pump manufacturer for any technical issues.

POSTOPERATIVE CONSIDERATIONS FOR AMBULATORY PERINEURAL CATHETERS

Ambulatory perineural catheters merit special considerations. Patients need to understand how to care for the insertion site, including the common possibility that the catheter may have some leakage. Patients need to understand that catheters can become inadvertently dislodged and be prepared for a backup pain management plan. Some practices allow patients to remove their own catheters if they are comfortable doing so.[25] No catheter should be removed while the limb is still insensate; if resistance or pain is experienced with catheter removal, patients should stop attempting to remove the catheter and seek medical attention. For patients whose catheters are difficult to remove, treatment strategies have been suggested, including obtaining a radiograph to ensure there is no knotting of the catheter, assessment with ultrasonography, applying gentle traction, and considering a surgical consult.[47,48] **Table 2** displays a sample of discharge instruction for ambulatory perineural catheters.

FUTURE CONSIDERATIONS

Setting up an ambulatory regional anesthesia program for orthopedic surgery can provide optimal perioperative anesthesia and analgesia, and can lead to greater patient satisfaction. With skilled practitioners and a streamlined system, efficiency can be preserved and even improved with faster PACU discharge. Future avenues in ambulatory regional anesthesia may include the development of newer techniques to extend the duration of analgesia provided by peripheral nerve blockade without unwanted side effects as well as multimodal regimens.

REFERENCES

1. Preti L, Senathirajah M, Sun C. Evaluation of the state ambulatory surgery databases, available through the HCUP central distributor, 2008. Healthcare cost and utilization project methods series report; 2011. Available at: http://www.hcupus.ahrq.gov/reports/methods/methods.jsp. Accessed April 15, 2014.
2. Barreveld A, Witte J, Chahal H, et al. Preventive analgesia by local anesthetics: the reduction of postoperative pain by peripheral nerve blocks and intravenous drugs. Anesth Analg 2013;116(5):1141–61.
3. Liu SS, Wu CL. The effect of analgesic technique on postoperative patient-reported outcomes including analgesia: a systematic review. Anesth Analg 2007;105(3):789–808.
4. Liu SS, Strodtbeck WM, Richman JM, et al. A comparison of regional versus general anesthesia for ambulatory anesthesia: a meta-analysis of randomized controlled trials. Anesth Analg 2005;101(6):1634–42.
5. Hanna MN, Murphy JD, Kumar K, et al. Regional techniques and outcome: what is the evidence? Curr Opin Anaesthesiol 2009;22(5):672–7.
6. Bingham AE, Fu R, Horn JL, et al. Continuous peripheral nerve block compared with single-injection peripheral nerve block: a systematic review and meta-analysis of randomized controlled trials. Reg Anesth Pain Med 2012;37(6):583–94.
7. Lehmann M, Monte K, Barach P, et al. Postoperative patient complaints: a prospective interview study of 12,276 patients. J Clin Anesth 2010;22(1):13–21.
8. Gan T, Sloan F, Dear Gde L, et al. How much are patients willing to pay to avoid postoperative nausea and vomiting? Anesth Analg 2001;92(2):393–400.
9. van den Bosch JE, Bonsel GJ, Moons KG, et al. Effect of postoperative experiences on willingness to pay to avoid postoperative pain, nausea, and vomiting. Anesthesiology 2006;104(5):1033–9.
10. Gan TJ, Diemunsch P, Habib AS, et al. Consensus guidelines for the management of postoperative nausea and vomiting. Anesth Analg 2014;118(1):85–113.
11. Memtsoudis SG, Ma Y, Swamidoss CP, et al. Factors influencing unexpected disposition after orthopedic ambulatory surgery. J Clin Anesth 2012;24(2):89–95.
12. Awad IT, Chung F. Factors affecting recovery and discharge following ambulatory surgery. Can J Anaesth 2006;53(9):858–72.
13. Brown AR, Weiss R, Greenberg C, et al. Interscalene block for shoulder arthroscopy: comparison with general anesthesia. Arthroscopy 1993;9(3):295–300.
14. Hadzic A, Arliss J, Kerimoglu B, et al. A comparison of infraclavicular nerve block versus general anesthesia for hand and wrist day-case surgeries. Anesthesiology 2004;101(1):127–32.
15. Hadzic A, Williams BA, Karaca PE, et al. For outpatient rotator cuff surgery, nerve block anesthesia provides superior same-day recovery over general anesthesia. Anesthesiology 2005;102(5):1001–7.
16. McCartney CJ, Brull R, Chan VW, et al. Early but no long-term benefit of regional compared with general anesthesia for ambulatory hand surgery. Anesthesiology 2004;101(2):461–7.
17. O'Donnell BD, Ryan H, O'Sullivan O, et al. Ultrasound-guided axillary brachial plexus block with 20 milliliters local anesthetic mixture versus general anesthesia for upper limb trauma surgery: an observer-blinded, prospective, randomized, controlled trial. Anesth Analg 2009;109(1):279–83.
18. Armstrong KP, Cherry RA. Brachial plexus anesthesia compared to general anesthesia when a block room is available. Can J Anaesth 2004;51(1):41–4.

19. Hadzic A, Karaca PE, Hobeika P, et al. Peripheral nerve blocks result in superior recovery profile compared with general anesthesia in outpatient knee arthroscopy. Anesth Analg 2005;100(4):976–81.
20. Williams BA, DeRiso BM, Engel LB, et al. Benchmarking the perioperative process: II. Introducing anesthesia clinical pathways to improve processes and outcomes and to reduce nursing labor intensity in ambulatory orthopedic surgery. J Clin Anesth 1998;10(7):561–9.
21. Gonano C, Kettner SC, Ernstbrunner M, et al. Comparison of economical aspects of interscalene brachial plexus blockade and general anaesthesia for arthroscopic shoulder surgery. Br J Anaesth 2009;103(3):428–33.
22. Ironfield CM, Barrington MJ, Kluger R, et al. Are patients satisfied after peripheral nerve blockade? Results from an International Registry of Regional Anesthesia. Reg Anesth Pain Med 2014;39(1):48–55.
23. Oldman M, McCartney CJ, Leung A, et al. A survey of orthopedic surgeons' attitudes and knowledge regarding regional anesthesia. Anesth Analg 2004; 98(5):1486–90 [table of contents].
24. Hofer J, Chung E, Sweitzer BJ. Preanesthesia evaluation for ambulatory surgery: do we make a difference? Curr Opin Anaesthesiol 2013;26(6):669–76.
25. Ilfeld BM. Continuous peripheral nerve blocks: a review of the published evidence. Anesth Analg 2011;113(4):904–25.
26. Lubarsky DA, Reves JG. Effect of subspecialty organization of an academic department of anesthesiology on faculty perceptions of the workplace. J Am Coll Surg 2005;201(3):434–7.
27. Carli F, Kehlet H, Baldini G, et al. Evidence basis for regional anesthesia in multidisciplinary fast-track surgical care pathways. Reg Anesth Pain Med 2011;36(1): 63–72.
28. Russell RA, Burke K, Gattis K. Implementing a regional anesthesia block nurse team in the perianesthesia care unit increases patient safety and perioperative efficiency. J Perianesth Nurs 2013;28(1):3–10.
29. Neal JM, Mulroy MF, Weinberg GL, American Society of Regional Anesthesia and Pain Medicine. American Society of Regional Anesthesia and Pain Medicine checklist for managing local anesthetic systemic toxicity: 2012 version. Reg Anesth Pain Med 2012;37(1):16–8.
30. Mariano ER. Making it work: setting up a regional anesthesia program that provides value. Anesthesiol Clin 2008;26(4):681–92, vi.
31. Gerancher JC, Viscusi ER, Liguori GA, et al. Development of a standardized peripheral nerve block procedure note form. Reg Anesth Pain Med 2005;30(1): 67–71.
32. Kinder R, Hsiung R. Overview of peripheral nerve blocks. In: Chu L, Fuller A, editors. Manual of clinical anesthesiology, vol. 1. Philadelphia: Wolters Kluwer Health/Lippincott Williams & Wilkins; 2012. p. 256–64.
33. Popping DM, Elia N, Marret E, et al. Clonidine as an adjuvant to local anesthetics for peripheral nerve and plexus blocks: a meta-analysis of randomized trials. Anesthesiology 2009;111(2):406–15.
34. Choi S, Rodseth R, McCartney CJ. Effects of dexamethasone as a local anaesthetic adjuvant for brachial plexus block: a systematic review and meta-analysis of randomized trials. Br J Anaesth 2014;112(3):427–39.
35. Desmet M, Braems H, Reynvoet M, et al. I.V. and perineural dexamethasone are equivalent in increasing the analgesic duration of a single-shot interscalene block with ropivacaine for shoulder surgery: a prospective, randomized, placebo-controlled study. Br J Anaesth 2013;111(3):445–52.

36. Katz J, Clarke H, Seltzer Z. Review article: preventive analgesia: quo vadimus? Anesth Analg 2011;113(5):1242–53.
37. Mercereau P, Lee B, Head SJ, et al. A regional anesthesia-based "swing" operating room model reduces non-operative time in a mixed orthopedic inpatient/outpatient population. Can J Anaesth 2012;59(10):943–9.
38. Friedman DM, Sokal SM, Chang Y, et al. Increasing operating room efficiency through parallel processing. Ann Surg 2006;243(1):10–4.
39. American Society of Anesthesiologists Task Force on Acute Pain Management. Practice guidelines for acute pain management in the perioperative setting: an updated report by the American Society of Anesthesiologists Task Force on Acute Pain Management. Anesthesiology 2012;116(2):248–73.
40. Usichenko TI, Rottenbacher I, Kohlmann T, et al. Implementation of the quality management system improves postoperative pain treatment: a prospective pre-/post-interventional questionnaire study. Br J Anaesth 2013;110(1):87–95.
41. Srikumaran U, Stein BE, Tan EW, et al. Upper-extremity peripheral nerve blocks in the perioperative pain management of orthopaedic patients: AAOS exhibit selection. J Bone Joint Surg Am 2013;95(24):e197(1–113).
42. Neal JM, Gerancher JC, Hebl JR, et al. Upper extremity regional anesthesia: essentials of our current understanding, 2008. Reg Anesth Pain Med 2009;34(2):134–70.
43. Alrajab S, Youssef AM, Akkus NI, et al. Pleural ultrasonography versus chest radiography for the diagnosis of pneumothorax: review of the literature and meta-analysis. Crit Care 2013;17(5):R208.
44. Enneking FK, Chan V, Greger J, et al. Lower-extremity peripheral nerve blockade: essentials of our current understanding. Reg Anesth Pain Med 2005;30(1):4–35.
45. Moore JG, Ross SM, Williams BA. Regional anesthesia and ambulatory surgery. Curr Opin Anaesthesiol 2013;26(6):652–60.
46. Williams BA, Kentor ML. The Wake(c) score: patient-centered ambulatory anesthesia and fast-tracking outcomes criteria. Int Anesthesiol Clin 2011;49(3):33–43.
47. Clendenen SR, Robards CB, Greengrass RA, et al. Complications of peripheral nerve catheter removal at home: case series of five ambulatory interscalene blocks. Can J Anaesth 2011;58(1):62–7.
48. Abrahams MS, Noles LM, Cross R, et al. Retained stimulating perineural catheters: a report of four cases. Reg Anesth Pain Med 2011;36(5):476–80.
49. Soares LG, Brull R, Lai J, et al. Eight ball, corner pocket: the optimal needle position for ultrasound-guided supraclavicular block. Reg Anesth Pain Med 2007; 32(1):94–5.

Perioperative Management of the Opioid Tolerant Patient for Orthopedic Surgery

Marchyarn Mahathanaruk, DO[a], James Hitt, MD, PhD[a],
Oscar A. de LeonCasasola, MD[a,b],*

KEYWORDS

- Opioid tolerance • Cellular mechanisms • Postoperative pain • Opioids • Ketamine

KEY POINTS

- Opioid tolerance may occur as early as 2 weeks after therapy is started with opioids.
- Patients who have received high doses of opioids preoperatively will respond better to therapy with opioids with high intrinsic efficacy, such as sufentanil.
- Evidence supporting the role of the N-methyl D-aspartate (NMDA) receptor in the development of tolerance suggests the use of NMDA receptor antagonists, such as ketamine, for the management of patients who are not responding to increasing doses of opioids.
- Epidural techniques with a local anesthetic and higher doses of morphine or sufentanil are effective in the management of postoperative pain in patients with opioid tolerance.

INTRODUCTION

Determining the number of patients with pain in the United States has been a difficult task, because calculations of the prevalence of pain vary depending on definitions of the levels of pain and methods used to quantify it. Recently, however, the Institute of Medicine (IOM) estimated that in 2011 there were 100 million individuals with pain in the United States.[1] This calculation was made based on a study that used a World Health Organization (WHO) World Mental Health Survey instrument in 10 developed countries and concluded that approximately 37% of adults have common chronic pain conditions.[1] It is noteworthy that these estimates do not include either patients with acute pain or children with pain. This increase in the prevalence of pain was paralleled by an increase in the use of prescription analgesics, including opioids. The National Health and Nutrition Examination Survey (NHANES) showed an increase in

[a] University at Buffalo Department of Anesthesiology, 252 Farber Hall, 3435 Main Street, Buffalo, NY 14214, USA; [b] Division of Pain Medicine, Department of Anesthesiology, Roswell Park Cancer Institute, Elm and Carlton Streets, Buffalo, NY 14263, USA
* Corresponding author. Division of Pain Medicine, Department of Anesthesiology, Roswell Park Cancer Institute, Elm and Carlton Streets, Buffalo, NY 14263.
E-mail address: oscar.deleon@roswellpark.org

Anesthesiology Clin 32 (2014) 923–932
http://dx.doi.org/10.1016/j.anclin.2014.08.009
anesthesiology.theclinics.com
1932-2275/14/$ – see front matter © 2014 Elsevier Inc. All rights reserved.

the number of Americans using opioids from the 1988 to 1994 period (3.2%) to the 2005 to 2008 period (5.7%).[1] Of these individuals, 7% were patients aged 65 years or older. Moreover, according to the White House Action Plan, the number of opioid prescriptions dispensed by retail pharmacies increased by 48%, representing 257 million prescriptions between 2000 and 2009.[2] Of the 3.61 billion total prescriptions filled in the United States in 2009, 7% were for opioids.[3] Clearly, opioid analgesic use among Americans, particularly individuals aged 65 years and older, has increased in the past 12 years. This increase in opioid use can be explained in part by the progressively increasing number of patients experiencing pain due to osteoarthritis, as members of the "baby boomer" generation have reached the age at which they begin to feel the effect of such conditions.[4]

A more cautious and thoughtful approach to opioid prescribing is further emphasized by the statistic that an estimated 35 million Americans have misused prescription opioids during their lifetimes, which translates to about 13.9% of the US population.[5] In 2011, 6.1 million Americans reported that they misused prescription opioids within the past month. Annual increases in prescription opioid misuse have been reported in all age groups, and an estimated 1.8 million people fit the criteria for substance abuse or dependence.[5] Moreover, recent pain therapy recommendations for geriatric patients suggest that the use of nonsteroidal anti-inflammatory drugs (NSAIDs) and cyclooxygenase-2 (COX-2) inhibitors may be associated with an increase in morbidity and mortality from cardiac and gastric causes, resulting in an increased reliance on opioid analgesics for pain treatment in these patients.[6]

To add an additional layer of concern, some data suggest that opioid therapy may not result in analgesic benefit and improved function in all patients suffering from osteoarthritis.[7] This recent systematic review of the use of traditional opioids in pain due to osteoarthritis concluded that this class of analgesics should not be used routinely for osteoarthritis.[7] This information suggests that practitioners should be very cautious when prescribing opioid analgesics and that patients receiving this class of analgesics should be continuously evaluated for therapeutic success as judged by pain and functionality improvement, side effects, adverse events, and aberrant behavior.[8] Treatment plans that include opioids should include an exit strategy concept,[9] whereby patients who do not show improvement in pain intensity and function after a reasonable opioid trial are quickly identified and titrated off opioid analgesics. This approach is not uniformly implemented by clinicians, and many patients who fail to respond to reasonable doses of opioids are placed on ever higher doses, increasing the risk of tolerance, opioid-induced hyperalgesia, and aberrant behaviors (misuse, abuse, and diversion).

Opioid-tolerant patients may present a significant problem for the management of postoperative pain, because patients who have received or self-administered opioids for as little as 2 weeks prior to surgery may exhibit signs of opioid tolerance, resulting in a higher perioperative opioid requirement.[10] This increased need for opioid medications may result in undertreatment, which can be misinterpreted as opioid craving or aberrant behavior. Moreover, the risk for physiologic withdrawal may also be present if their daily opioid consumption is abruptly decreased either because they failed to report their actual usage pattern or due to reluctance of health providers to match their preoperative dosing. This is particularly important in those patients who abuse opioids, because their daily opioid intake may be significantly greater than those patients taking them for therapeutic purposes. Moreover, the former patient population may also take other illicit drugs that may have effects on the N-methyl-D-aspartate receptor (NMDA) (eg, phencyclidine [PCP]) or combinations of this agent with other illicit drugs such as marijuana.[11]

Recent studies have helped elucidate the cellular mechanisms of opioid tolerance. This information has been useful in defining protocols for the management of patients with a history of high opioid intake so that these patients may also experience adequate postoperative pain control.

SUPRASPINAL MECHANISMS OF OPIOIDS

When opioids are administered via the oral or intravenous (IV) route, they bind the opioid receptors in the brainstem at the periaqueductal gray (PAG) region and the rostral ventromedial (RVM) nucleus. Neurons then project to the medullary reticular formation and the locus coeruleus (the major source of norepinephrine cells in the brain), probably through disinhibition, and inhibition of a tonically active inhibitory interneuron. These descending fibers, collectively known as the descending inhibitory pathways, comprise the dorsolateral funiculus in the spinal cord and project to the dorsal horn, where they synapse with the primary afferent neurons. These descending pain modulatory neurons release neurotransmitters in the spinal cord, especially serotonin (5HT) and norepinephrine (NE). The released NE and 5HT act to modulate the release of pain neurotransmitters, namely glutamate, substance P, calcitonin gene-related peptide, and brain-derived neurotrophic factor from the first order (presynaptic) neuron, and decrease the activation of the second-order neurons, namely the spinothalamic tract.[12]

CELLULAR MECHANISMS OF TOLERANCE

Opioid tolerance occurs as a result of quantitative and qualitative functional phenomena. Progressive loss of active receptor sites from prolonged agonist exposure may result in less fewer sites and decreased opioid analgesic action. Prolonged opioid exposure causes desensitization by uncoupling the opioid receptor from the guanosine triphosphate (GTP)-binding subunit, which decreases agonist-binding affinity.[13–15] This is because opioids inhibit adenylyl cyclase via a G_i protein mechanism, which decreases the synthesis of cyclic adenosine monophosphate (cAMP) (ie, a reduction in protein kinase A [PKA]-mediated phosphorylation of intracellular proteins).[16] This is, in fact, the underlying neurobiological mechanism by which opioids produce analgesia. However, in the face of opioid tolerance, intracellular cAMP returns to control levels, or may even be increased from the baseline. This is thought to be due to the uncoupling of the opioid receptor from the inhibitory G protein system.[17] Thus, the desensitization (a qualitative phenomenon) to agonist binding and the loss in the number of opioid receptors (a quantitative phenomenon) result in higher opioid requirements.

Trujillo and Akil[18] and Elliot and colleagues[19] have also implicated the NMDA receptor in the development of acute tolerance. Moreover, Mayer and colleagues[20] reported that opioid tolerance was associated with an increase in the second messenger protein kinase C (PKC), the production of nitric oxide (NO), and NO-activated poly-adenosine diphosphate (ADP) ribose synthetase (PARS)[21] activation within the superficial laminae of the dorsal horn. PKC has been shown to regulate the NMDA receptor through phosphorylation, which results in removal of a blocking magnesium ion.[22] This modulation of the NMDA receptor by PKC likely plays a key role in the development acute opioid tolerance. In fact, opioid tolerance in rodents can be inhibited by NMDA receptor antagonists, for example noncompetitive antagonists such as MK801, dextromethorphan, ketamine, and phencyclidine, and competitive NMDA receptor antagonists such as LY274614, NPC 17742, and LY235959.[23] Success has also been achieved with the use of partial glycine agonists (ACPC), glycine antagonists

(ACEA-1328), and nitric oxide synthase inhibitors (L-NNA, L-NMMA, and methylene blue.[23] A case report further suggests a for the NMDA receptor in opioid tolerance in people. The authors documented not only pain relief, but also a decrease in opioid requirements in a young patient with a history of heroin abuse after a suicide attempt that resulted in multiple traumatic injuries requiring T12-L1 spinal fusion. During the first 27 hours postoperatively, the patient required a total of 12 g of acetaminophen, 0.9 mg of clonidine, the patient's home dose of 40 mg of methadone, and up to 430 mg/d of IV morphine without improvement in her pain relief (visual analog scale [VAS], 5–7 out of 10). Ketamine infusion was started at 10 µg/kg/min and then was progressively reduced by steps of 2.5 µg/kg/min, over a period of 45 min, to a final dose of 2.5 µg/kg/min. Improvement in pain relief became evident in the first hour after the beginning of the ketamine infusion (VAS, 2 out of 10), and morphine consumption (patient-controlled analgesia) decreased to 160 mg/d. Ketamine was continued at 2.5 µg/kg/min until the fifth postoperative day and then again for 2 more days after the removal of misplaced screws. The VAS pain score remained at 3 out of 10 or below, and no neurologic sequelae were observed. Upon discharge, the patient left the hospital with a substitution treatment of 40 mg/d methadone.[24]

The potential use of ketamine in this setting is an important finding, as it has been shown that either a single dose or repeated administration of opioids may lead to activation of the NMDA receptor just as effectively as repeated C-fiber stimulation.[25,26] Thus, ketamine, as well as other NMDA receptor antagonists, could be useful in the treatment of acute postoperative pain in patients with opioid tolerance, as it not only reverses morphine tolerance and restores morphine effectiveness,[27] but it may also prevent the development of acute tolerance to opioids. An alternative, very exciting strategy is the use of benzamide, a selective PARS inhibitor that has been shown to reduce or even prevent the development of opioid analgesic tolerance and the resultant formation of dark neurons in adult male Sprague-Dawley rats.[21] Unfortunately, the development of benzamide has not progressed to human trials or usage to date.

The need to treat postoperative pain in patients with opioid tolerance is not only a clinical issue with moral and ethical implications, but also a neurobiological one. Uncontrolled pain produces morphologic changes in the receptive field zone of the spinal cord, leading to chronic pain patients using opioids to experience increased levels of postoperative pain that may result in both higher opioid requirements postoperatively and/or uncontrolled pain even in the face of the administration of increasing doses of opioids.[28] Thus, blockade of afferent pain signals before the nociceptive stimulus starts may be even more important in the chronic opioid user patient than in the opioid-naïve patient.[29]

BACKGROUND ON CLINICAL STUDIES

Clinical studies on opioid-tolerant patients are scarce. Moreover, the phenomenon of cross-tolerance between systemic and intraspinal opioids is a controversial issue due to the design of the studies that have evaluated this phenomenon. Although the authors,[30–32] as well as others[33] have published data to suggest that people experience cross-tolerance between the oral and intraspinal route, others have not shown the same results.[34,35] In the studies by Pfeifer[35] and Kossmann,[34] patients received 510 mg of epidural morphine and were followed for only 24 hours. Pharmacokinetic data show that high concentrations of morphine are achieved in both the lumbar and cervical cerebrospinal fluid (CSF) of patients receiving similar doses of morphine as those used in the studies by Pfeifer and Kossman 68 hours after lumbar epidural injection.[36] These high concentrations may saturate the opioid receptors acutely, masking any down regulation. Thus, cross-tolerance may not be evident after large epidural morphine doses, particularly when pain evaluation and opioid utilization analysis is limited to a 24-hour period. As the authors have documented in their studies,[30–32] patients with a history of opioid use not only require higher doses of opioids but also more days of therapy compared with opioid-naïve patients.

PROTOCOLS FOR PATIENT CARE IN THE POSTOPERATIVE PERIOD

The Division of Pain Medicine at Roswell Park Cancer Institute has used a multimodal protocol for the perioperative care of patients with a history of opioid use and clinical manifestations of opioid tolerance. The authors' approach includes the use of gabapentinoids and a selective NSAID.

Gabapentin is an antiepileptic medication that is known to modulate the release of excitatory neurotransmitters in the dorsal horn of the spinal cord by modulating the voltage-sensitive calcium channel. Gabapentinoids block this voltage-sensitive ion channel, causing a decreased influx of calcium and a reduced release of excitatory neurotransmitters into the synaptic cleft. In addition to this well-known property of gabapentinoids, they also have been shown to have supraspinal effects, enhancing the descending cortical inhibitory pathways by activating the α-2 adrenoceptor.[37] Treatment of rats with oral gabapentin increased concentrations of norepinephrine in the CSF and attenuated postoperative hyperalgesia in a dose-dependent fashion. This effect of gabapentin pretreatment was blocked with specific α-2 receptor antagonists.[38] Gabapentin has also been studied in people, and a meta-analysis examined 12 randomized controlled studies and reported reduced pain intensity scores (at 4 hours and 24 hours) and reduced opioid consumption in the immediate postoperative period.[39] Pregabalin and gabapentin have a similar mechanism of action, but pregabalin has better bioavailability and penetration into the central nervous system. A prospective, randomized, controlled trial of pregabalin (preoperative dose of 300 mg followed by a 2-week tapering dose schedule) showed reductions in perioperative opioid consumption and a reduced incidence of persistent neuropathic pain at 3 months and 6 months.[40] Preoperative celecoxib has also been shown to reduce postoperative pain intensity and to reduce postoperative opioid requirements in a dose-dependent fashion.[41] The analysis showed that 400 mg of preoperative celecoxib prolonged the time to rescue medication use compared with placebo (6.6 hours vs 2.3 hours), reduced the need for rescue medication in the first 24 hours (63% vs 91%), and did not change the adverse event incidence.[41]

If there is a contraindication to the implementation of a perioperative regional anesthesia technique, or the site of surgery is not amenable for this type of therapy, IV patient-controlled analgesia (PCA) is utilized. A basal infusion can be calculated based on the patient's baseline 24-hour opioid utilization. For this purpose, the authors calculate that a daily dose of 90 mg of oral morphine, 60 mg of oral methadone, 45 mg of oral oxycodone, 12 mg of oral hydromorphone, or 25 µg/h of transdermal fentanyl is equivalent to 2 to 3 mg of IV hydromorphone or 2 to 4 µg/h of IV sufentanil.[42] IV breakthrough doses of 20% of the basal infusion dose of hydromorphone or sufentanil are also prescribed. The patient is evaluated every 6 hours after the PCA infusion has been started, and the doses of hydromorphone or sufentanil are adjusted to limit the number of breakthrough boluses to 2 to 3 per hour. In patients with cancer-related pain, acetaminophen (APAP) has been shown to decrease opioid requirements and improve pain and wellbeing in patients treated with moderate doses of opioids.[43] Moreover, Sinatra and colleagues[44] showed that patients undergoing hip and knee arthroplasties who were treated with IV APAP differed significantly from the placebo group in pain relief from 15 minutes to 6 hours ($P<.05$) and the median time to morphine rescue, 3 hours versus 0.8 hours. IV APAP also reduced morphine consumption over the 24-hour period, 38 plus or minus 35 mg versus 57 plus or minus 2.3. This represents a 33% (about 19 mg) reduction in morphine consumption. Consequently, the authors routinely use IV APAP in these patients and convert them to oral dosing as soon as they tolerate oral feedings.

Another adjuvant that the authors use in these patients is IV dexamethasone. A meta-analysis of 24 randomized clinical trials by De Oliveira and colleagues[45] that included 2751 subjects showed that the mean (95% confidence interval [CI]) combined effects favored dexamethasone over placebo for pain at rest (≤4 h, −0.32 [0.47 to −0.18], 24 h, −0.49 [−0.67 to −0.31]) and with movement (≤4 h, −0.64 [−0.86 to −0.41], 24 h, −0.47 [−0.71 to −0.24]).[45] Moderate doses (0.11–0.2 mg/kg) and high doses (>0.21 mg/kg) of dexamethasone decreased opioid consumption to a similar extent (−0.82 [−1.30 to −0.42] and −0.85 [−1.24 to −0.46]), respectively, but there was no benefit with low doses (<0.1 mg/kg). No increase in analgesic effectiveness or reduction in opioid use could be demonstrated between the high- and intermediate-dose dexamethasone. Preoperative administration of dexamethasone appears to produce a more consistent analgesic effect compared with intraoperative administration. They concluded that IV dexamethasone at doses of 0.2 mg/kg is an effective adjunct in multimodal strategies to reduce postoperative pain and opioid consumption after surgical procedures. In the opioid-tolerant patient, dexamethasone is particularly effective, because it both decreases the presynaptic release of neurotrasmitters,[46] and the production of kynurenic acid, an NMDA antagonist.[46,47] Because opioid tolerance may be associated to NMDA receptor activation, dexamethasone may contribute to improve analgesia in these patients by these aforementioned mechanisms. The authors recommend administering a loading dose of 20 mg intravenously and then continue therapy with 8 mg intravenously every 6 hours for 8 days. A proton pump inhibitor is always used, and therapy is discontinued by weaning dexamethasone over an additional 8-day period. If adequate pain control is not achieved despite these strategies, a continuous infusion of ketamine is started at 5 μg/kg/min and then titrated up by 1 μg/kg/min every 8 to 12 hours to achieve a balance between analgesia and side effects, which frequently include diplopia, sedation, and dizziness and analgesia. In the face of these side effects, the authors stop further increases in the doses of ketamine for 24 hours, and then try to increase them as noted. The use of bolus loading dose of ketamine is discouraged, because it is frequently associated with bad dreams and hallucinations.

Patients treated with epidural anesthesia and analgesia received bolus doses of 5–10 mL of 0.5% ropivacaine before the surgical incision was made. A continuous infusion of 0.5% ropivacaine and 0.013% MS (4 mg of morphine in 30 mL of ropivacaine) was then started at 4–6 mL/h and titrated according to hemodynamic response. Postoperatively, patients received a continuous epidural infusion of 0.2% ropivacaine + 0.02% MS at 2 to 4 mL/h. Breakthrough doses of 2 mL every 10 minutes were provided. If dynamic pain control (VAPS <4/10 during movement) was not achieved within 1 hour, the infusion rate was increased by 1 mL every hour.

Most patients can be managed this way but will require 8 to 10 days of therapy if infusions are only decreased by 1 mL/h when the VAPS have remained below 4/10 for 6 consecutive hours.[32] Conversely, if pain control is not achieved despite adjustments in the basal infusion up to 5 mL/h, morphine is replaced by sufentanil. The new solution (0.2% ropivacaine + 0.0002% [2 μg/mL] sufentanil) is infused at 2 to 3 mL/h, and breakthrough doses of 2 mL every 10 minutes are provided. The basal infusion is titrated every hour to maintain a dynamic VAPS less than 4/10. In this way, patients with severe opioid dependency have been managed successfully at the authors' institution.[30,31]

Drug tolerance at the spinal level is characterized as being time-[48] and dose-dependent.[49] Opioid-tolerant patients experience more effective analgesia at lower doses during frequently adjusted continuous infusions (IV, epidural, or perineural) compared with larger intermittent bolus dosing.

Finally, in the authors' experience, the use of epidural opioid analgesia was associated with both excellent pain control in opioid-tolerant patients and the prevention of physiologic opioid withdrawal symptoms.[30–32] This phenomenon is probably because of relatively high concentrations of opioids in the cisterna magna and the limbic system, thus halting the development of withdrawal, despite significant vascular uptake and supraspinal redistribution seen with sufentanil following epidural administration.[31] Opioid-tolerant patients receiving perineural local anesthetic infusions are still at risk for opioid withdrawal, so home doses of oral opioids can be given or converted to equivalent IV doses until oral intake can resume.

SUMMARY

In the future, patients with opioid tolerance will be managed with multimodal anesthetic strategies that result in blockade of afferent signals followed by postoperative administration of opioids with high intrinsic efficacy, NMDA receptor antagonists, and PKC, NO, and PARS inhibitors.

REFERENCES

1. Institute of Medicine Committee on Advancing Pain Research, Care and Education, The National Academies Collection. Reports funded by National Institutes of Health. Relieving pain in America: a blueprint for transforming prevention, care, education, and research. Washington, DC: National Academies Press (US) National Academy of Sciences; 2011.
2. White House Commission on Complementary and Alternative Medicine Policy. March 2002. U.S. Government Printing Office. Washington DC. http://www.whccamp.hhs.gov/. Accessed September 23, 2014.
3. National Association of Chain Drug Stores. 2009 community pharmacy results. 2009. Available at: http://www.nacds.org/user-assets/pdfs/.../2008Community PharmacyResults.pdf. Accessed March 9, 2012.
4. Hootman JM, Helmick CG. Projections of US prevalence of arthritis and associated activity limitations. Arthritis Rheum 2006;54(1):226–9.
5. U.S. Department of Health and Human Services, Substance Abuse and Mental Health Services Administration, Center for Behavioral Health Statistics and Quality, editors. Results from the 2011 National Survey on Drug Use and Health. Rockville (MD): Research Triangle Institute; 2011. Available at: http://www.samhsa.gov/data/NSDUH/2011SummNatFindDetTables/Index.aspx.
6. American Geriatrics Society Panel on Pharmacological Management of Persistent Pain in Older Persons. Pharmacological management of persistent pain in older persons. J Am Geriatr Soc 2009;57(8):1331–46.
7. Nuesch E, Rutjes AW, Husni E, et al. Oral or transdermal opioids for osteoarthritis of the knee or hip. Cochrane Database Syst Rev 2009;(4):CD003115.
8. de Leon-Casasola OA. Opioid therapy in 2012: a call for a high degree of attention to detail. Introduction. J Pain Symptom Manage 2012;44(Suppl 6):S1–3.

9. Ballantyne JC, Mao J. Opioid therapy for chronic pain. N Engl J Med 2003; 349(20):1943–53.

10. Twycross RG. Choice of strong analgesic in terminal cancer: diamorphine or morphine? Pain 1977;3(2):93–104.

11. Administration D.E. Phencyclidine. 2013. Available at: http://www.deadiversion.usdoj.gov/drug_chem_info/pcp.pdf. Accessed September 16, 2014.

12. Vanderah TW. Pathophysiology of pain. Med Clin North Am 2007;91(1):1–12.

13. Chavkin C, Goldstein A. Reduction in opiate receptor reserve in morphine tolerant guinea pig ilea. Life Sci 1982;31(16–17):1687–90.

14. Chavkin C, Goldstein A. Opioid receptor reserve in normal and morphine-tolerant guinea pig ileum myenteric plexus. Proc Natl Acad Sci U S A 1984;81(22):7253–7.

15. Rogers NF, el-Fakahany E. Morphine-induced opioid receptor down-regulation detected in intact adult rat brain cells. Eur J Pharmacol 1986;124(3):221–30.

16. Guitart X, Nestler EJ. Identification of morphine- and cyclic AMP-regulated phosphoproteins (MARPPs) in the locus coeruleus and other regions of rat brain: regulation by acute and chronic morphine. J Neurosci 1989;9(12):4371–87.

17. Cox B. Molecular and cellular mechanisms in opioid tolerance. In: Besson J, Basbaum AI, editors. Towards a New Pharmacotherapy of Pain. Chichester (United Kingdom): John Wiley and Sons Ltd; 1991. p. 135–56.

18. Trujillo KA, Akil H. Inhibition of morphine tolerance and dependence by the NMDA receptor antagonist MK-801. Science 1991;251(4989):85–7.

19. Elliott K, Minami N, Kolesnikov YA, et al. The NMDA receptor antagonists, LY274614 and MK-801, and the nitric oxide synthase inhibitor, NG-nitro-L-arginine, attenuate analgesic tolerance to the mu-opioid morphine but not to kappa opioids. Pain 1994;56(1):69–75.

20. Mayer DJ, Mao J, Price DD. The development of morphine tolerance and dependence is associated with translocation of protein kinase C. Pain 1995;61(3):365–74.

21. Mayer DJ, Mao J, Holt J, et al. Cellular mechanisms of neuropathic pain, morphine tolerance, and their interactions. Proc Natl Acad Sci U S A 1999;96(14):7731–6.

22. Chen L, Huang LY. Protein kinase C reduces Mg2+ block of NMDA-receptor channels as a mechanism of modulation. Nature 1992;356(6369):521–3.

23. Herman BH, Vocci F, Bridge P. The effects of NMDA receptor antagonists and nitric oxide synthase inhibitors on opioid tolerance and withdrawal. Medication development issues for opiate addiction. Neuropsychopharmacology 1995; 13(4):269–93.

24. Haller G, Waeber JL, Infante NK, et al. Ketamine combined with morphine for the management of pain in an opioid addict. Anesthesiology 2002;96(5):1265–6.

25. Larcher A, Laulin JP, Celerier E, et al. Acute tolerance associated with a single opiate administration: involvement of N-methyl-D-aspartate-dependent pain facilitatory systems. Neuroscience 1998;84(2):583–9.

26. Mao J, Price DD, Mayer DJ. Mechanisms of hyperalgesia and morphine tolerance: a current view of their possible interactions. Pain 1995;62(3):259–74.

27. Shimoyama N, Shimoyama M, Inturrisi CE, et al. Ketamine attenuates and reverses morphine tolerance in rodents. Anesthesiology 1996;85(6):1357–66.

28. Dubner R. Pain and hyperalgesia following tissue injury: new mechanisms and new treatments. Pain 1991;44(3):213–4.

29. Woolf CJ. Recent advances in the pathophysiology of acute pain. Br J Anaesth 1989;63(2):139–46.

30. de Leon-Casasola OA, Lema MJ. Epidural sufentanil for acute pain control in a patient with extreme opioid dependency. Anesthesiology 1992;76(5):853–6.

31. de Leon-Casasola OA, Lema MJ. Epidural bupivacaine/sufentanil therapy for postoperative pain control in patients tolerant to opioid and unresponsive to epidural bupivacaine/morphine. Anesthesiology 1994;80(2):303–9.
32. de Leon-Casasola OA, Myers DP, Donaparthi S, et al. A comparison of postoperative epidural analgesia between patients with chronic cancer taking high doses of oral opioids versus opioid-naive patients. Anesth Analg 1993;76(2):302–7.
33. Muller H, Stoyanov M, Borner U. Epidural opiates for relief of cancer pain. In: Yaksh TL, Müller H, editors. Spinal opiate analgesia: experimental and clinical studies. Berlin (NY): Springer-Verlag; 1982. p. 147, xii.
34. Kossmann B, Dick W, Bowdler I. Modern aspects of morphine therapy. In: Wilkes E, Napp Laboratories, editors. Advances in morphine therapy: International congress and symposium series/Royal Society of Medicine. London: Royal Society of Medicine; 1984. p. 73–85.
35. Pfeifer BL, Sernaker HL, Ter Horst UM, et al. Cross-tolerance between systemic and epidural morphine in cancer patients. Pain 1989;39(2):181–7.
36. Brose WG, Tanelian DL, Brodsky JB, et al. CSF and blood pharmacokinetics of hydromorphone and morphine following lumbar epidural administration. Pain 1991;45(1):11–5.
37. Gee NS, Brown JP, Dissanayake VU, et al. The novel anticonvulsant drug, gabapentin (Neurontin), binds to the alpha2delta subunit of a calcium channel. J Biol Chem 1996;271(10):5768–76.
38. Hayashida K, DeGoes S, Curry R, et al. Gabapentin activates spinal noradrenergic activity in rats and humans and reduces hypersensitivity after surgery. Anesthesiology 2007;106(3):557–62.
39. Hurley RW, Cohen SP, Williams KA, et al. The analgesic effects of perioperative gabapentin on postoperative pain: a meta-analysis. Reg Anesth Pain Med 2006;31(3):237–47.
40. Buvanendran A, Kroin JS, Della Valle CJ, et al. Perioperative oral pregabalin reduces chronic pain after total knee arthroplasty: a prospective, randomized, controlled trial. Anesth Analg 2010;110(1):199–207.
41. Derry S, Moore RA. Single dose oral celecoxib for acute postoperative pain in adults. Cochrane Database Syst Rev 2013;(10):CD004233.
42. de Leon-Casasola O. Implementing therapy with opioids in patients with cancer. Oncol Nurs Forum 2008;35(Suppl):7–12.
43. Stockler M, Vardy J, Pillai A, et al. Acetaminophen (paracetamol) improves pain and well-being in people with advanced cancer already receiving a strong opioid regimen: a randomized, double-blind, placebo-controlled cross-over trial. J Clin Oncol 2004;22(16):3389–94.
44. Sinatra RS, Jahr JS, Reynolds LW, et al. Efficacy and safety of single and repeated administration of 1 gram intravenous acetaminophen injection (paracetamol) for pain management after major orthopedic surgery. Anesthesiology 2005; 102(4):822–31.
45. De Oliveira GS Jr, Almeida MD, Benzon HT, et al. Perioperative single dose systemic dexamethasone for postoperative pain: a meta-analysis of randomized controlled trials. Anesthesiology 2011;115(3):575–88.
46. Hong D, Byers MR, Oswald RJ. Dexamethasone treatment reduces sensory neuropeptides and nerve sprouting reactions in injured teeth. Pain 1993;55(2): 171–81.
47. Marek P, Ben-Eliyahu S, Vaccarino AL, et al. Delayed application of MK-801 attenuates development of morphine tolerance in rats. Brain Res 1991;558(1): 163–5.

48. Wiesenfeld Z, Gustafsson LL. Continuous intrathecal administration of morphine via an osmotic minipump in the rat. Brain Res 1982;247(1):195–7.
49. Stevens CW, Monasky MS, Yaksh TL. Spinal infusion of opiate and alpha-2 agonists in rats: tolerance and cross-tolerance studies. J Pharmacol Exp Ther 1988;244(1):63–70.

SUGGESTED READING

Carroll IR, Angst MS, Clark D. Management of perioperative pain in patients chronically consuming opioids. Reg Anesth Pain Med 2004;29:576–91.

Index

Note: Page numbers of article titles are in **boldface** type.

Anesthesiology Clin 32 (2014) 933–941
http://dx.doi.org/10.1016/S1932-2275(14)00122-0
1932-2275/14/$ – see front matter © 2014 Elsevier Inc. All rights reserved.

anesthesiology.theclinics.com

United States Postal Service

Statement of Ownership, Management, and Circulation
(All Periodicals Publications Except Requestor Publications)

1. Publication Title		2. Publication Number							3. Filing Date
Anesthesiology Clinics		0	0	0	-	2	7	7	9/14/14

4. Issue Frequency	5. Number of Issues Published Annually	6. Annual Subscription Price
Mar, Jun, Sep, Dec	4	$313.00

7. Complete Mailing Address of Known Office of Publication (*Not printer*) (*Street, city, county, state, and ZIP+4®*)

Elsevier Inc.
360 Park Avenue South
New York, NY 10010-1710

Contact Person
Stephen R. Bushing

Telephone (*Include area code*)
215-239-3688

8. Complete Mailing Address of Headquarters or General Business Office of Publisher (*Not printer*)

Elsevier Inc., 360 Park Avenue South, New York, NY 10010-1710

9. Full Names and Complete Mailing Addresses of Publisher, Editor, and Managing Editor (*Do not leave blank*)

Publisher (*Name and complete mailing address*)

Linda Belfus, Elsevier Inc., 1600 John F. Kennedy Blvd., Suite 1800, Philadelphia, PA 19103-2899

Editor (*Name and complete mailing address*)

Pamela Hetherington, Elsevier Inc., 1600 John F. Kennedy Blvd., Suite 1800, Philadelphia, PA 19103-2899

Managing Editor (*Name and complete mailing address*)

Adrianne Brigido, Elsevier Inc., 1600 John F. Kennedy Blvd., Suite 1800, Philadelphia, PA 19103-2899

10. Owner (*Do not leave blank. If the publication is owned by a corporation, give the name and address of the corporation immediately followed by the names and addresses of all stockholders owning or holding 1 percent or more of the total amount of stock. If not owned by a corporation, give the names and addresses of the individual owners. If owned by a partnership or other unincorporated firm, give its name and address as well as those of each individual owner. If the publication is published by a nonprofit organization, give its name and address.*)

Full Name	Complete Mailing Address
Wholly owned subsidiary of	1600 John F. Kennedy Blvd, Ste. 1800
Reed/Elsevier, US holdings	Philadelphia, PA 19103-2899

11. Known Bondholders, Mortgagees, and Other Security Holders Owning or Holding 1 Percent or More of Total Amount of Bonds, Mortgages, or Other Securities. If none, check box ☐ None

Full Name	Complete Mailing Address
N/A	

12. Tax Status (*For completion by nonprofit organizations authorized to mail at nonprofit rates*) (*Check one*)
The purpose, function, and nonprofit status of this organization and the exempt status for federal income tax purposes:
☐ Has Not Changed During Preceding 12 Months
☐ Has Changed During Preceding 12 Months (*Publisher must submit explanation of change with this statement*)

PS Form 3526, August 2012 (Page 1 of 3 (Instructions Page 3)) PSN 7530-01-000-9931 PRIVACY NOTICE: See our Privacy policy in www.usps.com

13. Publication Title			14. Issue Date for Circulation Data Below
Anesthesiology Clinics			September 2014

15. Extent and Nature of Circulation			Average No. Copies Each Issue During Preceding 12 Months	No. Copies of Single Issue Published Nearest to Filing Date
a. Total Number of Copies (*Net press run*)			842	927
b. Paid Circulation (By Mail and Outside the Mail)	(1)	Mailed Outside-County Paid Subscriptions Stated on PS Form 3541. (*Include paid distribution above nominal rate, advertiser's proof copies, and exchange copies*)	353	378
	(2)	Mailed In-County Paid Subscriptions Stated on PS Form 3541 (*Include paid distribution above nominal rate, advertiser's proof copies, and exchange copies*)		
	(3)	Paid Distribution Outside the Mails Including Sales Through Dealers and Carriers, Street Vendors, Counter Sales, and Other Paid Distribution Outside USPS®	197	219
	(4)	Paid Distribution by Other Classes Mailed Through the USPS (e.g. First-Class Mail®)		
c. Total Paid Distribution (*Sum of 15b (1), (2), (3), and (4)*)		▲	550	597
d. Free or Nominal Rate Distribution (By Mail and Outside the Mail)	(1)	Free or Nominal Rate Outside-County Copies Included on PS Form 3541	100	105
	(2)	Free or Nominal Rate In-County Copies Included on PS Form 3541		
	(3)	Free or Nominal Rate Copies Mailed at Other Classes Through the USPS (e.g. First-Class Mail)		
	(4)	Free or Nominal Rate Distribution Outside the Mail (Carriers or other means)		
e. Total Free or Nominal Rate Distribution (Sum of 15d (1), (2), (3) and (4))		▲	100	105
f. Total Distribution (Sum of 15c and 15e)		▲	650	702
g. Copies not Distributed (See instructions to publishers #4 (page #3))		▲	192	225
h. Total (Sum of 15f and g)		▲	842	927
i. Percent Paid (15c divided by 15f times 100)		▲	84.62%	85.04%

16. Total circulation includes electronic copies. Report circulation on PS Form 3526-X worksheet.

17. Publication of Statement of Ownership
If the publication is a general publication, publication of this statement is required. Will be printed in the **December 2014** issue of this publication.

18. Signature and Title of Editor, Publisher, Business Manager, or Owner

[signature] Stephen R. Bushing – Inventory Distribution Coordinator

Date September 14, 2014

I certify that all information furnished on this form is true and complete. I understand that anyone who furnishes false or misleading information on this form or who omits material or information requested on the form may be subject to criminal sanctions (including fines and imprisonment) and/or civil sanctions (including civil penalties).

PS Form 3526, August 2012 (Page 2 of 3)

Moving?

Make sure your subscription moves with you!

To notify us of your new address, find your **Clinics Account Number** (located on your mailing label above your name), and contact customer service at:

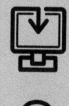

Email: journalscustomerservice-usa@elsevier.com

800-654-2452 (subscribers in the U.S. & Canada)
314-447-8871 (subscribers outside of the U.S. & Canada)

Fax number: 314-447-8029

Elsevier Health Sciences Division
Subscription Customer Service
3251 Riverport Lane
Maryland Heights, MO 63043

*To ensure uninterrupted delivery of your subscription, please notify us at least 4 weeks in advance of move.

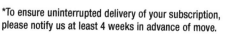

Printed and bound by CPI Group (UK) Ltd, Croydon, CR0 4YY

03/10/2024

01040489-0019